"*The Harm We Do* is a welcome and important contribution to the field of medical ethics. Dr. Poole is an impassioned advocate of both medicine and the church. She knows and loves her church, knows and cherishes the ability of modern medicine to enrich the lives of her patients, and finds herself torn by the conflicts and misunderstandings between her two loves.

"Dr. Poole writes eloquently and with familiarity with church doctrine and with modern science. But one is impressed more by her compassion than by her knowledge. As she describes a case history, one senses that she shares the pain and fear of the patient, and that her decision will come not on the basis of 'What does the church command?' or 'What do my colleagues recommend?' but by asking, 'What is the most human thing that can be done here?' Wise and loving books like this one are rare in the field of medical ethics, and we are fortunate to have this one."

Rabbi Harold S. Kushner
Author, *When Bad Things Happen to Good People*

"...an eminently readable and exquisitely sensitive book in medical ethics. *The Harm We Do* is presented in a format which is reflective, contemplative, even prayerful. One comes away from it with an increased awareness of the grandeur of the human and of the awesome responsibilities shouldered by the members of the health care profession.

"Fully aware and respectful of the Catholic church's official positions in matters of the new reproductive technologies, Dr. Poole raises important questions and is not afraid to respectfully dissent. This she never does without first reflecting deeply on the situation from her moral, medical, and faith perspectives. Though not always able to come to definitive answers in these complicated matters, she consistently demonstrates just how a believer ought to go about making a right moral decision. This book is a valuable resource for all engaged in health care and health care ethics."

Dick Westley
Author, *Good Things Happen*
Life, Death, and Science

"I wish this book had been available during the 30 years I practiced and taught family planning. Not only would it have supported my own convictions, but it would have helped the clinic staff, trainees, and students, and provided great comfort to those patients struggling to reconcile the teaching of the church with the realities of their daily lives and moral judgment.

"This is not a book to sit on the shelves of reference libraries. It should be available in every general practice and family planning clinic as well as being essential reading for the clergy and policy makers in the developing world."

Nancy B. Loudon

Heal

D1397435

"Dr. Poole writes with wisdom and experience. She recalls older Catholic teaching on sex as dour and heartless, especially toward women. She worries that official Catholic moral teaching today has become excessively detailed, leaving little room to individual judgment in differing circumstances. She provides helpful summaries of pertinent medical information on what once seemed to be settled matters, such as conception, which many now understand as a process rather than a moment. The implications of this new view for moral judgments about the status of the human embryo is stimulating and controverted.

"This book ranges widely, asking many pointed questions and offering the views of a conscientious Catholic physician on many of them. This is a book that will stir discussion. Along with the inevitable heat, I hope the discussion will produce needed light for the church the author loves."

John P. Boyle, Ph.D.
Professor, School of Religion
University of Iowa

"*The Harm We Do* is a frank, documented discussion of the moral values championed by the Catholic church in all phases of medical ethics. Well written, with courageous honesty, the book confronts the dilemma faced by the conscientious Catholic between contemporary scientific experience and ideological Vatican pronouncements. Although reflecting the British environment, Dr. Poole respects the American nuances in ethical perceptions. She is an excellent guide to the ideal and the pragmatic in Christian ethical values."

F.X. Murphy, C.SS.R. (Also known as Xavier Rynne)
Professor Emeritus, Academia Alfonsiana, Rome

"In *The Harm We Do* Dr. Joyce Poole provides the most knowledgeable, balanced, and lucid account of Catholic and non-Catholic concerns and perspectives with respect to family planning that I have read. With delicate and compassionate skill, she applies a wealth of scientific facts and extensive clinical experience so as to enable readers to make wise choices when confronted with some of life's most difficult decisions. This book will enable persons of diverse religious belief to find considerable common ground in the field of reproductive morality."

R.T. Ravenholt, M.D.
Director, World Health Surveys, Inc.

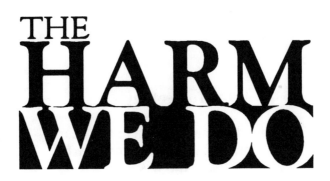

THE HARM WE DO

A Catholic Doctor Confronts
Church, Moral, & Medical Teaching

JOYCE POOLE

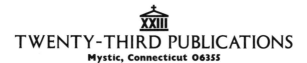

XXIII
TWENTY-THIRD PUBLICATIONS
Mystic, Connecticut 06355

To Geoffrey

Indeed you love truth in the heart;
Then in the secret of my heart
teach me wisdom.

Psalm 50

Twenty-Third Publications
185 Willow Street
P.O. Box 180
Mystic CT 06355
(203) 536-2611
800-321-0411

ISBN 0-89622-543-7
Library of Congress Catalog Card Number 92-82673

PREFACE

So many friends and one-time colleagues have given freely of their time and specialized fields of knowledge that it would be invidious to try to name them all. I hope they will accept this inclusive expression of my great indebtedness.

My deepest thanks, however, must be expressed to Dr. Christopher Cameron who has read each section with enthusiasm and meticulous care; his concern for sense and language has prevented many an inaccuracy or ambiguity. Any that remain are, of course, my own.

I sincerely thank Celina Bullick as well, whose intelligent deciphering of the manuscript and accurate typing made the production of the original book both a possibility and a pleasure.

FOREWORD

As a committed Christian and Catholic, Dr. Joyce Poole tries to live out her faith in her daily life. All of us committed believers strive to have our faith permeate all that we do, and we are constantly aware of the problems and difficulties faced in the process. Dr. Poole confronts a special problem in her daily life. As a Catholic physician, she disagrees with some of the specific teachings of the hierarchical magisterium on medical ethics. In fact, in her judgment these teachings actually harm people.

Writing out of her British perspective and context, the author discusses the same specific issues that American Catholic physicians face. Her religious faith, honesty, common sense, matter-of-fact approach, obvious commitment to her patients, and sensitive knowledge of medicine come through on every page. American Catholic physicians, health care professionals, and hospital chaplains as well as Catholic hierarchical teachers and ethicists need to listen to this voice, even if they do not agree with all that is said.

The traditional first principle of medical morality maintains that no harm should be done. Joyce Poole has come to the conclusion that some Roman Catholic hierarchical teachings do cause harm.

In my judgment as a Catholic moral theologian, Dr. Poole appeals to a very fundamental and distinctive characteristic of Catholic moral theology to disagree with some of the more specific teachings of the hierarchical magisterium.

The Catholic moral tradition to its great credit has insisted on what is called an intrinsic morality. What does it mean to say that morality is intrinsic? Too many people think of morality as some-thing imposed on us from the outside. The Catholic approach, however, insists that morality involves what is good for the human person; morality and the truly human are identical. St. Thomas Aquinas, the most significant figure in the Roman Catholic theological tradition, develops his whole ethical system in the light of this intrinsic approach. While emphasizing the importance of human fulfillment and happiness, Aquinas and the Catholic approach reject any individualism that sees the person as existing by oneself isolated from all others. Morality consists in what is truly good for the human person existing in the midst of significant relationships with God, neighbor, world, and self.

But what about natural law? Has natural law not been the approach associated with Aquinas and the Roman Catholic tradition? Law by its very nature seems to imply something imposed from without. Such is not the understanding of law in the Thomistic and Catholic traditions. The best of the natural law tradition maintains that human reasoning reflecting on human nature can discover what is truly human behavior. Two characteristics of this approach deserve further scrutiny.

The first characteristic understands law in general and the natural law in particular as an ordering of reason. Most people automatically think of law as an act of the will of the legislator telling somebody what is to be done. If law is an act of will, something is good because it is commanded. If law is an ordering of reason, then something is commanded because it is good. The natural law in the best of Catholic tradition involves an intrinsic approach to morality: something is commanded because it is good for the person.

A second important characteristic of Catholic natural law concerns its meditational or participative nature. One Thomistic description understands natural law as the participation of eternal law in the rational creature. The eternal law constitutes the plan of God for the world. Reason, reflecting on the human nature that God has created, can come to understand this plan of God which calls for what is ultimately both to the glory of God and to the happiness and fulfillment of human beings.

I strongly support this fundamental perspective that insists on an intrinsic morality, but I disagree about aspects of the meaning of human nature and reason as found in the teaching of the hierarchical magisterium. Dr. Poole implicitly follows the same approach.

Not all Roman Catholics share the position of Dr. Poole and myself that the hierarchical teaching on some specific moral issues is wrong, but we who take such a position must try to understand what has happened. How and why has the hierarchical magisterium come to specific moral teachings that seem to go against the fundamental Catholic assertion that morality involves doing what is for the good of the person?

Dr. Poole does not directly address this much discussed question, but she occasionally refers to two very important emphases on the teaching of the hierarchical magisterium that have contributed to the present problem: authoritarianism and the tendency to give too much certitude to teaching on very specific issues.

In the light of Dr. Poole's book and some of the remarks she makes, the Catholic emphasis on an intrinsic approach to morality helps us to recognize the aberration of authoritarianism and to envision how the hierarchical teaching office should function. The hierarchical teaching office does not make a moral teaching right or wrong. Something is taught because it is right, and not the other way around. The hierarchical teaching office itself must constantly search for moral truth and wisdom.

A second reason why many Catholics, who agree with the basic Catholic presupposition about intrinsic morality, disagree about some specifics comes from the claim of the hierarchical magisterium to have too great a certitude about very specific and complex moral issues. Poole hints at this many times in this book. Logic requires that the more specific and the more complex the issue, the harder it is to claim a certitude that excludes all possibility of error. All can agree with great certitude that murder is always wrong, but heated discussion often occurs in discussing whether or not certain acts of killing may be accepted (e.g., capital punishment, war). Too often today the hierarchical magisterium claims too great a certitude for its teaching on specific and complex moral issues.

Dr. Poole writes as a very competent and committed physician who is a loyal Roman Catholic. As a Catholic moral theologian, I do not agree with all her particular positions in this book, but the church as a whole needs this open, frank, and charitable discussion so that the teaching of the hierarchical magisterium will be what is truly for the good of human persons and their communities.

Perhaps the greatest problem we face as a church catholic today concerns the matter of unity and diversity within the church. The tone and the content of this book well exemplify what we as a church catholic strive to live: in necessary matters, unity; in doubtful matters, freedom; in all matters, charity.

Charles E. Curran
Elizabeth Scurlock University Professor of Human Values
Southern Methodist University

From a Medical Doctor

FOREWORD

In her book, *The Harm We Do: A Catholic Doctor Confronts Church, Moral, and Medical Teaching*, Dr. Joyce Poole vividly brings out the painful quandaries shared by many Catholics, including many physicians, on the subjects of authority, suffering, contraception, sterilization, fertility, abortion, homosexuality, AIDS, transplant surgery, death and dying, and other areas affected by the moral position of the Catholic church.

For one thing, she became a Catholic in her adult years when the church was undergoing profound changes in the aftermath of the historical Second Vatican Council. For another, she is well aware that the church's stand on many of these issues is related to "interfering with nature." But Poole also contends that it is of the essence of medical science itself to interfere with nature. Moreover, both her professional training and the oaths she took as a doctor of medicine oblige her to serve people who are in need of medical care, including the areas covered by her church's teachings.

Confronted by the unrelenting stand of the church on various aspects of these issues, especially contraception, sterilization, and the deadly disease called AIDS, Dr. Poole stands by her personal and compassionate convictions. She finds that the teachings of Vatican II stand by her on the matter.

> Every man has the duty and therefore the right to seek the truth in matters religious in order that he may with prudence form for himself right and true judgments of conscience with the use of all suitable means (*Dignitatis Humanae*, par. 3).

All the faithful, clerical and lay, possess a lawful freedom of inquiry and thought and the freedom to express their minds humbly and courageously about those matters in which they enjoy competence *(Gaudium et Spes,* par. 62).

And that is exactly what Dr. Poole does: express her mind humbly but courageously about those matters she enjoys competence in by virtue of her being an informed Catholic and a physician with years of experience, including surgery, obstetrics, and gynecology. She is, by her own definition, a Catholic who "finds Christ's continuing presence in the church and its sacraments, rather than a member of a sect that has singular and often perplexing views on certain aspects of sexual and medical ethics." Her book reflects her own view and, in effect, the views of some Catholic bishops' conferences "that there is more than one way of looking at moral problems within the framework of sincere Christian conviction."

One such way is the traditional "formula" way, which older and more traditional Catholics sincerely espouse, namely, "What does the book say?" The other is the way of Vatican II- oriented Catholics: the conscientious way of personally reviewing "what the book says" in the light of newfound knowledge and newly encountered situations, and what the Spirit of Christ urges in their situation.

The first way is more akin to the dependent certitude of a child who looks to rules for security; the second, the prudential certitude of a mature adult who realizes that ultimately the God-given responsibility to act on any matter is his or hers alone. To quote Dr. Poole: "Rules offer a security that most people at times would prefer to responsibility, but there is a danger of producing a person who in Mark Twain's words is "'good in the worst sense of the word.'"

As a Catholic, Dr. Poole respects but does not deify rules. As a physician, she also respects but does not deify traditional medical teachings. Rather, she situates them in the context of what the truth-up-to-the-present (what others would term the present state of the art) reveals, leaving room for other dimensions of truth as they emerge or are discovered. In her own words, "Religion is concerned with ultimate questions, and advances in medicine force it to question ultimate aims."

This is, I believe, the power of this book. It is in its own way personally religious, but not dogmatic; it is scientific, but does not deify science; respects technological innovations, but does not submit itself to the impositions of what some people call technocracy. Religion, science, and technology are always placed in the service of humankind.

Dr. Poole airs very timely appeals to two kinds of people most involved with patients, especially on the matter of contraception, sterilization, AIDS, and abortion. To the physicians, she appeals for competence and care. To priests, for compassion and understanding. To both, utmost care so that too paternalistic an approach might not become to patients-penitents a "disabling substitute" for the more difficult task of ordering their own lives.

Although people are becoming better informed in the areas of medicine and religion, Dr. Poole rightly cautions both doctors and clerics to continue to be most careful in their areas of care. "Misguided spiritual advice or a harsh judgment made of a penitent can cause in a sensitive person a loss of self-esteem from which he or she may never recover. Similarly, a wrong interpretation by a physician of a single abnormality can cripple the patient not only physically but emotionally as well." Indeed, as Dr. Poole says, the responsibility on the shoulders of those who deal with people in trouble is a heavy one. Thus it is good that neither the doctor or the priest is any longer regarded as if he or she were God.

Finally, many of the dilemmas she discusses in her book "have resulted from comparatively recent medical advances, each of which has raised a new set of moral problems to which there are no ready answers." Dr. Poole forewarns and thus forearms the Christian doctor to always "be prepared to carry the cross of uncertainty when trying to balance the claims of the patient's needs against those arising from his or her concept of traditional Christian moral norms and against the specific teaching of the magisterium of the church."

As a Catholic and medical practitioner, I share Dr. Poole's painful dilemma. Like her, I have many times in the past carried "the cross of uncertainty," always invoking the help of the Holy Spirit to liberate my patients from any of my own human deficiencies. Indeed, this is often the only way medical doctors can avoid the greater harm they might otherwise inflict on their patients!

Juan M. Flavier, M.D., M.P.H.
Secretary of Health
Republic of the Philippines

CONTENTS

INTRODUCTION

...the dialogue between bio-ethics and belief must be pursued in order to bring a deeper awareness of what really constitutes that love of neighbor or quest for human betterment upon which each is engaged.[1]

Many in the Western world see the Catholic church as being in a state of decline that is approaching crisis. Priests are dying or leaving the church in greater numbers than they are being ordained, and the numbers of practicing Catholic laity have fallen dramatically. Whatever the causes might be, it is essential in such a setting that the truths the church proclaims and represents are not obscured by irrelevancies and inessentials. A Catholic is a person who finds Christ's continuing presence in the church and its sacraments, rather than a member of a sect that has singular and often perplexing views on certain aspects of sexual and medical ethics.

This book is mainly about these non-essential issues. It reflects on the fact that there is more than one way of looking at moral problems within the framework of sincere Christian conviction.

While it is an accepted legal maxim that hard cases make bad law, it is my experience as a Catholic doctor that in the moral field, especially that of medical ethics, there is no general precept so determinate that it can be applied with confidence to all particular cases. I fear, for those of us within the church, that too much specific moral direction in this area by the magisterium might endanger its credibility and authority on more important matters central to its teaching. It would be a matter of great concern if we were to end up with a code of ethics out of touch with the body of the church.

Within the Catholic church nothing can have caused more widespread and unprecedented dismay than the publication in 1968 of *Humanae Vitae,* Pope Paul VI's encyclical on birth control. Since then, to those outside it, the image of the church has been distorted by an apparent obsession with sexual ethics.

I came into the church in the wake of the encyclical, having been many years on the way and after instruction from several priests of different backgrounds. I knew I did not agree with the church's stand on contraception and saw this as a possible though not central problem. During my instruction period the subject was never mentioned; my instructors also regarded the matter as peripheral to the core of Catholic Christian belief.

A high and informed standard of ethical behavior is not, of course, a Christian prerogative. It has been specifically demanded of physicians since the early Greeks, and is enshrined both in the law and requirements of medical organizations.

Furthermore, it is generally understood that Catholic and other Christian moral teaching relies on reason as well as authority, and the churches have grown historically by learning from the prudent judgment of their members. In the past, pronouncements on subjects as diverse as Darwinism and slavery have had to be adjusted to keep pace with scientific and social progress.

When the teaching of the church on ethical matters is out of tune with human perception and medical experience, a real conflict is set up within many of us who would count ourselves as committed Catholics. It is the theme of these reflections that the best that many of us can do is to carry the burden of uncertainty willingly, and if possible cheerfully, as part of our human condition, trusting that in the final analysis we are judged not by our mistakes but by our intentions.

Chapter 1

REFLECTIONS ON AUTHORITY

We all like rules; in childhood, indeed, our security depends on them. The child of the overstrict parent may envy his friend whose mother is ever indulgent, but both are immeasurably more fortunate than the one whose parents have no consistent rules at all, who is allowed to do something one day and not the next. We cannot grow up and mature, unfortunately, without leaving behind such childhood certainties, but the hankering for them remains. We like to know where we are. In illness and in old age we see how quickly people become hospitalized and institutionalized; rules designed mainly for safety and smooth running are quickly seized upon by people too frail to be burdened with choice or responsibility.

In the Catholic church, with a tradition of authority stronger than most, older people still remember wistfully their younger days when rules and sins were more clearly defined, and life was, or so it was thought, correspondingly easier. Rules offer a security that most people would at times prefer to responsibility, but there is a danger of producing a person who in Mark Twain's words "is good in the worst sense of the word."

It must be right that the Second Vatican Council (1962-1965) should have changed the focus.

> ...every man has the duty, and therefore the right, to seek the truth in religious matters, in order that he may with prudence form for himself right and true judgments of conscience, with the use of all suitable means.[1]
> ...all the faithful, clerical and lay, possess a lawful freedom

of inquiry and thought, and the freedom to express their minds humbly and courageously about those matters in which they enjoy competence.[2]

In the Church of England, *The Family in Contemporary Society*, a report to the Lambeth Conference of Bishops in 1958, attempted to apply the method of interdisciplinary study and discussion in such a way that "theological insights were allowed to illuminate and articulate the moral claim inherent in the subjects under discussion, without dictating prior conclusions."[3] The church seemed to be acknowledging that in a time of rapid advances in so many scientific fields they did not always have at hand the solution to all particular problems.

In the field of medical ethics these problems have increased exponentially since the documents were written. Reproductive techniques then unthought of have become attainable; the contraceptive pill has become easily obtainable and widely used; transplant surgery of vital organs is commonplace. Sophisticated rescuscitative procedures for the desperately ill and for the grossly premature baby can no longer be included in the term "extraordinary means," traditionally used by the church. When, the practicing doctor might ask, do the means required to keep someone alive become "extraordinary," or when, for that matter, does a "brain-dead" patient stop being "someone"? If the state of not-yet-being-someone exists and can be defined, should the embryo too be legitimately available for biological research in the service of others? The Catholic church emphatically forbids the last, while most others, including the Episcopal church of England, are less certain.

Progress in reproductive techniques such as *in vitro* fertilization, together with understanding and overcoming some of the most common causes of infertility, depend on the availability of spare embryos for research purposes. These include failure of the fertilized ovum to develop or implant itself, together with the large problem of male infertility. The use of embryos for research is widely accepted by the other mainstream churches and by the public at large, and the Catholic church, if it is to avoid the label of a sect, will have to define its position coherently and rationally rather than present it as a set of deeply held convictions.

The singling out by the magisterium of the Catholic church of moral issues concerned with sexual and reproductive functions has almost certainly caused more perplexity than any other issue for those both inside and outside its fold. Although many guidelines and directives have been issued, there can be no field wider than bioethics where the exceptional case so often presents itself, not so much as a matter for discussion between moral theologians, but as a position to be taken in the face of urgent human problems. In the 1950s, Situation Ethics drew strong condemnation from Pope Pius XII. This has since been upheld, yet is not ethics intimately concerned with what to do when you are not sure what to do?[4] It is one thing in a doctrinal context and by appeal to tradition and natural law to argue a case against contraception, for example, but quite another to refuse help, either clinically or pastorally, to a woman distraught with too much childbearing. Such a woman may be incapable of understanding or applying so-called natural methods and may well have a husband who would not cooperate if she did. The Catholic doctor might have to choose between upholding the moral dogma of the church and helping his patient. E.M. Forster, the English novelist, famously remarked that if he had to choose between betraying his friend and betraying his country, he hoped he would have the courage to betray his country.

Christianity is not a system of ethics, though it adds another dimension to decision making. It will not tell us what to do, though belief and grace may increase our moral insight and enable us to see more clearly and act, if necessary, more courageously. A moral person in either the secular or Christian sense will have no real problem in deciding between good and bad. The difficulty is between good and good, or bad and bad, and most real moral problems in daily life fall into this category. Such moral decisions are as often as not about who is to get hurt, and the injunction to love everybody does not help, although it is frequently invoked by religious people. The trouble with Situation Ethics, of course, is that it does not really help where help is most needed. It is easier to agree to the commandment to love one's neighbor than to decide who that neighbor is. Religion is concerned with ultimate questions, and advances in medicine force it to question ultimate aims.[5] Religion and medicine are traditionally associated from the ancient world through Judaism and Christianity, but the principles of the first applied to the second do not necessarily lead to detailed conclusions reaching through the whole field of medical ethics and pastoral counseling.

The commandment to remember the Sabbath and keep it holy had to do with not working for a time and making time and space for God; it had little to do with the minutiae of Jewish law in the time of Jesus—who did not hesitate to say so—or with the austerities of Sunday in some of the strictly Sabbatarian Western Islands of Scotland. In the same way, it seems probable that the commandment "Thou shalt not kill" should be interpreted not so much as a rule to be applied, say, to the early embryo, but as a directive to be *concerned* about killing, whether directly and intentionally, or indirectly and unintentionally by poverty, famine, or the pollution of the environment in the cause of profit and greed.

If it is accepted that no precept of law, civil or ecclesiastic, can possibly determine the values to be considered and balanced in every particular case, we are thrown upon our own appraisal of the situation and an awareness of the touchstones in our lives that give a sense of what comes from God.

> Conscience is the most secret core and sanctuary of a man. There he is alone with God, whose voice echoes in his depths.... To obey [his conscience] is his very dignity: according to it he will be judged.[6]

Since the documents of the Second Vatican Council were written, many will consider that the church has moved back from this focus on the supremacy of conscience to the pre-conciliar emphasis on directives and authority. I have heard *Gaudium et Spes* ruefully translated as Some Hope and No Joy.

Without questioning the authority of the magisterium of the church in matters within its competence, there is an authority too residing in those of us who have a lifetime of listening in close and frank contact to the problems of ordinary people. We must be ready to accept that we may make a decision that involves the cross: criticism, self-doubt, or censure. In the physician's office or in the confessional, human decisions must, nevertheless, be made. After considering all the factors, including the teaching of the church, we may judge that ultimately three persons matter: ourselves, God, and the patient.

Chapter 2

Reflections on Suffering

"No one could believe in God and work here."

This comment was made by a senior nurse in the children's hospital where we had both worked for some years. It was an acute surgical ward, and it was Christmas Day, which made the circumstances memorable. The convalescent children were singing carols and enjoying hilarious games while a little boy, admitted that day from a road accident, died quietly behind screens. We had to take off our party hats to attend to him. In an inconspicuous corner was a two-year-old girl with such appalling congenital facial deformities that an official visitor that morning had literally fainted at the sight of her. We were trying to improve surgically the worst of her malformations, but she would provoke horror and pity for the rest of her life.

The paradox of an all-powerful yet all-loving God, apparently passive in the face of human suffering, is to many people the main objection to Christian belief.[1] It would seem that a choice would have to be made between all-powerful and all-loving, or more easily, to retreat altogether into agnosticism. Those whose daily work brings them into intimate contact with suffering and death—nurses, doctors, clergy—must perhaps, more urgently than most, come to a working philosophy of suffering in the context of their religious belief.

Does God actually *will* suffering? Many Christian people seem to believe, implicitly at least, that God does. "It is hard to see God's will in this," they will say. It seems that many religious people have made the underlying assumption that their pain or bereavement is indeed the will of God, perplexing though it might be. Had the child dying behind the screens been "called to a higher life," as would no doubt be said later by somebody at his funeral, or had he simply been in the way of a car driven by someone who had had too much to drink over Christmas? Had the girl with the facial deformity been singled out in some way by a God who could see some ultimate good come out of it, or was she the victim of a chance throw of the genetic dice?

It has to be remembered, of course, that chance genetic variation can work for good and give us a Mozart or an Einstein, and it is almost certainly the mechanism of natural selection. If so, what is God's role as creator of all things, including the very substance of genes? These are big questions, and although big answers will not be attempted here, an effort must be made if a working faith is to be woven into a working life, and if there is to be some kind of wholeness of outlook.

In this century, advances in the basic sciences have demonstrated a chaos and apparent randomness in the realms of particle physics and biology; this is some distance removed from the comparatively simple cause-and-effect, or "clockwork," image of matter and the universe, which was the legacy of Newtonian physics. Nonetheless, there is, in the natural creation, a system of physical laws that remain constant and predictable and without which our experience of life would be chaotic. If one could not depend, say, on the unvarying operation of the laws of gravity, then walking, eating, and even digestion would be difficult and the safe landing of an airliner impossible. If a stone, obeying these constant laws, falls from a high building and kills an unfortunate person in the street, do we see it as God's direct will that it should fall just there, and if it is not, can God suspend that particular law momentarily "like some Divine laser beam," as the Anglican Bishop of Durham puts it? If God can, and does not, it is hard to see God as the loving father of the gospels, who cares for each one of us and for the sparrows too.

At a lenten discussion group in a parish the subject of destiny came up. All (except myself) contended that if I were to be killed in an accident on my way home they would see it as God's will that my life should end that night, that it would all be part of a divine plan. Had I shared this view and, driving home without care and attention killed some pedestrian, would that also have been seen as God's plan? What if the person had not been killed, but brain damaged, and they and their family suffered greatly for the rest of their lives? The argument can be extended indefinitely, but in that direction lies madness, and this could not lead to a Christian view of life. It is a kind of thinking common in wartime when people will say in an air-raid that a bomb will not fall on you unless it has your name on it. If it has, that's it. If it hasn't, you are safe. It is a comfortable philosophy in time of danger, popular in the trenches of the First World War, but not easily credible.

What then of natural disasters, which undoubtedly cause suffering? Perhaps if the crust of Earth were of uniform thickness and density earthquakes as such would not occur and we should have no recurring disasters. Earthquakes, like floods and plague, are often listed by insurance companies as "acts of God."

Bacteria, viruses, and DNA molecules are part of a balanced ecology obeying biophysical laws within an orderly creation. Without bacteria to break down dead matter, Earth would be choked with dead things. If these bacteria, following their own intrinsic nature like the stone falling from the building, invade living tissue and cause disease, can we again expect God to intervene specifically in the ecological system and change the principles of cellular metabolism and reproduction on which our whole biological system depends? Death, it has been said, is a biological necessity, and God made creation the way it is.

Lead can be a deadly poison and has been shown beyond reasonable doubt to cause central nervous system damage in children who have lived in areas of high traffic density. This is surely our fault when we fail so miserably to reduce the source of contamination rather than God's fault for making the intrinsic properties of lead. Lead is "good" when it is used as a shield against x-rays.

Malignant disease is an abnormality of cellular division which is not yet fully understood, though it is clear that it can be caused by some irritants, a few of which have been identified. It has been postulated that some degenerative diseases of the central nervous system may have an environmental factor. We are still probably at an early stage of human development in understanding, adapting to, and protecting our environment.

What though of pain? Of course it is protective, warning us of disease and injury, but could not God have devised a less "painful" method of protecting us? So often it appears to have no useful function. Once a bone is broken it seems a pity that it goes on hurting. The problem is that pain-carrying nerve fibers, which we regard as "good" when they warn us of trouble in a tooth, are designed specifically to carry pain. If we demand that they transmit instead warm comfortable feelings, it would be asking God to change their very nature; it would be like asking lead not to act like lead when it gets into the central nervous system, but to act dependably like lead when it is used as a screen to protect radiologists from harmful exposure to x-rays.

We have our God-given intelligence as well as the resources to prevent much suffering. We know more or less where earthquake zones are, where rainfall is likely to fail, where population growth is exceeding the food supply, and how to prevent much disease. If we fail to apply our knowledge through lack of will or from material greed, it seems unfair to regard the resultant suffering as "acts of God." I doubt if prayers for rain in Africa, however sincerely made, are ever *directly* answered by climatic change. But God moves in mysterious ways. Bob Geldof, the Irish pop-singer, was himself a kind of miracle when he single-handedly raised so much help for famine relief in Ethiopia in 1984. God seems to prefer to act through people.

When pain occurs, doctors are highly privileged in often having the means to relieve it. Pain clinics are available in most major hospitals, and highly sophisticated techniques are being rapidly developed for the relief of intractable pain, such as can occur in bone. The Hospice Movement, with its expert management of terminal pain, graces our society.

It is not denied for a moment, of course, that good can come out of suffering. People can rise to heroic heights in dealing with personal or social catastrophe, and thereby gain in spiritual growth and insight. At such times most of us hope for the loving support of family and friends, and this can be the source of much of our strength. Those who love us suffer with us, not able to bear our pain physically, but suffering nonetheless. Daniel Berrigan, S.J., tells a moving story of his own near-death experience in a prison hospital. He asks himself afterward if in this he had seen God's face. No, he had not, he thought. Then on further reflection, yes he had, in the presence and anxious faces of those who loved him and upheld him in the long hours. Is this not what we ask of God?[2]

The centrality of a suffering God distinguishes Christianity from other mainstream religions. Can a transcendent God suffer? If Jesus Christ, God Incarnate as we believe, showed us what God was like, then suffering was part of his revelation. His passion occurred at a historical point in time, but that bit of God that we could witness could be likened to the rings in the trunk of a tree, visible only where they are exposed but running down to the roots of the past and into the branches of the future.[3] The incarnation showed us perhaps not only what God was like but enabled God to know what it was like to be us: to suffer pain, fear, loneliness, and abandonment not only by his friends but by the Father. "My God, why have you forsaken me?" Anything we go through, God has gone through. Of course, God cannot share physical suffering with us now, but the loving-father image is central to Christian belief. The suffering of loving parents for their children is part of human experience. We create our children, love them, and bring them up in accordance with our own principles: if they suffer physically, or hurt one another, or let us down, we

suffer for them and with them. The pain of anxiety about someone we love is hard to locate or to describe, but we know it because we experience it.

"Clinical detachment" is often described as a virtue to be cul-
tivated in doctors. I have reservations about this. Some self-
discipline is necessary, of course, for psychological health and to
preserve the ability to carry on professionally, but I believe the
good doctor must accept to some extent the burden of in-
volvement. As Carl Rogers maintains, the medical professional
must go further than seeming to care; he must actually care.[4] To
allow patients to share their suffering, fear, and grief in this way
is neither unrealistic nor self-righteous; it is no more than God
asks us to do as members of the mystical body: God's hands, feet,
words. If we are aware of the presence of God in our daily work
we can make emergency contact. "Lord, help me to be patient
with this tiresome woman." "God, help me to be calm in this
alarming situation so that I may do my best." It doesn't always
work; irritation may get the upper hand, and the desperately ill
patient may die, but help has come in the asking.

Clinical detachment has its place in another sense, and a very
important one. The doctor or other professional care-giver must
be able to withdraw when his services are no longer needed. Our
ultimate aim is to help people to do without us.

Dr. Robert Runcie (Archbishop of Canterbury, 1980-1990)
translates Emmanuel Kant's "wonder at the moral law within"
less imposingly as "wonder at the fact that things matter."[5]

To return to the nurse at the children's hospital. An awareness
that things matter is present in most people even if it is un-
acknowledged and unexpressed, and whether or not they sub-
scribe to a formal religious belief. It is almost certainly the basis of
the human ability to work and survive in the face of great suffering and overwhelming adversity.

Chapter 3

CONTRACEPTION

However much the church may idealize family life, there seems to be little doubt that it has a considerable distaste for sex.

The association of women with uncleanliness predates Christianity, of course, and has been a facet of many cultures, including that of the Jews in the time of Jesus. Strict rules were devised for the segregation of menstruating women within the family and within society. The woman in Mark's gospel who had an issue of blood for twelve years was suffering from more than her bleeding; she was also a social outcast and unclean. School girls still refer to the "curse," and the Episcopal church had until fairly recently at least a service for the "churching" of women after childbirth, liturgically a thanksgiving, but more often regarded by the people as a kind of ritual cleansing before being received back into the Christian community. One of my grandmothers (a devout Protestant), still adhering to the old requirement of the penitentials and ancient moral teaching, would not partake of Holy Communion when she was menstruating; the other grandmother would not make jam or butter at that time, since she believed that they would not keep.

If the traditional Christian view of women and sexuality has its roots in the Genesis account of Adam and Eve, the theology of sexual activity as sinful was suggested by Paul who observed, in advising married couples about their mutual sexual rights, that he was writing by way of "forgiveness" (concession), not of command.[1]

Three centuries later, Augustine concluded that if there was scope for forgiveness, then there must be something culpable connected even with Christian marital sexual activity. It was in sexual arousal that he experienced and observed the most blatant instance of that law of sin in his body on which he found St. Paul so enlightening.[2] Augustine's disgust with sexuality has colored church thinking ever since. It is recorded that at his conversion in 386 when he heard a divine voice directing him to the Scriptures he at once lighted upon the passage, "Put on the Lord Jesus Christ and make not provision for the flesh and the lusts thereof." Although it was he who articulated the classic moral principle that a good end never justifies evil means, he writes, on the question of sexuality, "He who has lawful intercourse through shameful lust is putting something evil to good use,"[3] and "What father would agree to hand his daughter over to the lust of another man, were it not for children?"[4] If lawful marital sexual activity was considered in this light, it is not difficult to see how the church's teaching on contraception evolved; it would allow us the sin without the excuse. The procreation of children was the only possible justification for indulging in an activity that was at best a distasteful duty and at worst, disgusting.

This distaste for sexuality almost certainly influenced the church's elevation of the state of virginity and priestly celibacy. The insistence on the perpetual virginity of Mary is a point of difference between the Roman and the Orthodox churches. The reformed churches do not seem to worry about it one way or the other.

On a visit to Jerusalem I heard an Armenian Christian guide refer to James, "brother of Our Lord," as the founder of his church. The following day another guide, presumably Roman Catholic, declared that such people were clearly greatly in error since it is known "as a fact" "that Mary was forever virgin." In his opinion, therefore, their church was built on a false premise, making any thought of future intercommunion out of the question.

In the second century the book of James elaborated various versions of the early life of Mary. One theory was that she was the second wife of Joseph, having been previously his ward. James by this reckoning could have been an earthly "half" brother of Jesus, a tortuous compromise perhaps, but one that underlines the intrinsic value attached by the church to physical virginity and that unfortunately obscures the *theological* significance of the virginal conception of Jesus.

Celibacy can be strongly defended, of course, on grounds other than the negative virtue of sexual continence. The word is given two shades of meaning in the *Oxford English Dictionary*: to refrain from sexual activity, and to live unmarried. The second aspect frees the priest and religious from all the secondary consequences of the married state: the provision of shelter, food, and education for wife and children, and from the social responsibilities of an extended family. This makes possible an immensely valuable gift to the life of the church in the form of freedom and single-minded devotion to the service of God. Cardinal Hume of Westminster put it vividly and simply on a television program. He was spending Saturday evening at a youth club in his diocese and one of the children asked him why he wasn't married. "Well," he said, "if I were married I would be spending the evening at home with my wife and family, and instead I am here with you."

The ban on contraception within marriage was dropped by the bishops of the Church of England in 1930, but it continues in the Catholic church to this day. In 1968 the reaffirmation of this traditional doctrine by Pope Paul VI in the encyclical *Humanae Vitae* burst upon the post-conciliar church like a bombshell. Many, if not most, ordinary Catholics in those heady years thought they could consign the church's teaching on birth control to a place in history. In the often over-large Catholic families of their youth the constant anxiety about yet another pregnancy had been a nightmare that mothers did not want their daughters to inherit: the physical and mental harm done to women by the church's restrictions on birth control is incalculable. There had been so much lightening of the load of traditional doctrines about sin and hell that many presumed the condemnation of birth control to have gone too.

Until 1950 even periodic abstinence had been firmly condemned as frustrating the basic function of marriage. Catholics since then have been cleared for "natural" methods of contraception. This of course effectively allows separation of the marital act from the possibility of procreation, so denying the very core of the church's teaching, namely, that human intercourse should always be open to the transmission of life. Catholics who use the "safe period" do so precisely because they hope to avoid this possibility, and the concession signified a major change.

Many people thereafter found it hard to see any difference *in principle* between one method of birth control and another. The contraceptive pill was generally understood to have been within a hairbreadth of being accepted by the Vatican. In 1963, shortly before he died, Pope John XXIII set up a commission to study the problem of overpopulation in the light of the church's teaching on birth control. As it soon became clear that the underlying basic issue was the church's whole stance on marital sexuality, the commission was enlarged to include doctors, sociologists, theologians, diocesan priests, and lay representatives. Sixty-four of its members eventually voted to drop the ban and four voted to retain it.

I think it is accepted that many left the church for good, no longer able to reconcile its teaching on this issue with the realities of their own daily lives and moral judgment. Most of those who remained seemed to have decided to follow their own consciences in this matter, while remaining faithful to what they considered to be the church's central doctrines. They saw the minutiae of the teaching on birth control by Rome as an intrusion on their marriage and as an unseemly irrelevance. The reaction of many moral theologians to the papal statement was the first significant dissent to Roman moral teaching in 200 years.

When the disciplinary moves against Charles Curran came to a head in 1986, I was interested and surprised at the amount of coverage the media gave it. Program followed program with interviews and discussion and it was very clear what the American Catholic laity thought. Curran, at least on the contraceptive issue, was expressing the views already held and followed by a huge majority. Most of them regarded the issue as long dead.

The Contraceptive Pill

As a Catholic doctor, I have had a close and privileged view of Catholic thinking on contraception over many years, and in this time the clinical scene has changed completely.

The contraceptive pill was licensed for use in the United States in 1959 and in Britain two years later. In the 1960s, Catholic patients were coming to ask me for the pill because they had heard that it "regulated the periods." I would agree that this was so and would explain the mechanism and pharmacology. The original estrogenic pill acted by suppressing ovulation completely, and as a result, there was less build-up of the endometrial lining of the uterus. The subsequent "period"—which is in reality withdrawal bleeding—was regular, slight, and usually painless; this made it a valuable and recognized treatment for heavy bleeding or period pains. In the absence of any medical contra-indication, the patient would usually decide to try it, and so the little deception would be innocently established between us and continue over the years. The word "contraception" hung between us unexpressed; the principle of double effect is well recognized in Catholic moral theology. One Catholic patient told me with unconscious humor that she was "taking it religiously."

Some of the later, predominantly progestogenic, pills do not interfere with ovulation, but act by making the cervical mucus impenetrable to sperm and the endometrium inimicable to implantation, should fertilization, by any chance, occur. This last possibility has led to the charge that such pills are potentially abortifacient which, in the strictly biological sense of preventing further development, is patently true. In practice, those Catholic doctors who hold this view and are vehemently opposed to this type of pill are unlikely in any case to prescribe any form of contraceptive, while those Catholic patients who come for contraceptive advice are, in my experience, either uninterested in or unconcerned about the difference. Believing that patients should be treated as responsible people, I would try to explain, as far as it could be explained and understood, the mode of action of any drug prescribed, whether it was for contraception or cardiac failure. In this matter, however, patients had for the most part already made up their minds.

Both the short- and long-term side effects of the contraceptive pill are so widely reported in the general press that with an increasingly well-informed laity we have people who have themselves weighed the acceptable risks and advantages before coming for advice. The pill has, of course, in addition to its perceived simplicity and reliability, an enormous esthetic advantage; the taking of it is separated from the context in which it acts and it is, furthermore, in the hands of the woman, which is a very important consideration in many marriages.

In Britain in the early years, the pill, if it was to be used for purely contraceptive purposes, had to be written as a private prescription which was paid for by the patient at the pharmacy. If it was prescribed for primarily medical reasons, such as excessive or painful menstrual bleeding, it could be written on a National Health Service form like any other medicine and was therefore free. Small statutory charges have now been introduced in the UK for other drugs and appliances, but prescriptions for contraceptives are exempt. Which form to use was often a difficult decision affecting the patient's sensibilities more importantly than her purse. It was a minefield through which one just had to pick one's way, using tact and empathy rather than the rule book.

Over the next 20 years the picture changed completely. Patients who were pillars of the church, bringing up their children in the faith and helping with parish activities, would come and ask straight out for the pill or for other contraceptive advice. It was tacitly assumed that I, as a Catholic doctor, would have no hesitation in advising on the matter.

I too, of course, had read *Humanae Vitae,* and understood, and indeed shared, Pope Paul's disquiet at the effect of too easily available contraception. The easier sexual morality that has become the norm would seem at first sight to bear witness to his perception, yet I am unconvinced that the two are so clearly related. Historically and geographically, sexual behavior has varied enormously from one generation to another and from one class or culture to another quite independently of contraceptive availability. Consider only that girls are reaching physical maturity earlier than their mothers and grandmothers, while at the same time their schooling has extended further into the teens. Girls and boys who have reached puberty in the first or second year of high school are still behind their desks when sexuality is at its height. (Let us remember that Romeo and Juliet were reputed to have been 14.) Social mores too, whether sex, alcohol, or smoking, are hugely influenced by the media, which are now penetrating our lives on an unprecedented scale.

It would seem that moral, social, and psychological attitudes have more bearing on extramarital sexual activity than the availability of effective contraception. This activity is, however, not necessarily promiscuous. In a study in Britain three-fifths of the sexually experienced had had only one partner, and half of those who had had intercourse intended to marry their partner.[5]

In a small-town environment where the standard of living may be quite high and free of inner-city anonymity, schoolgirls are by no means lining up for prescriptions for the pill. There are some, of course, but invariably they are those who are already leading an active sexual life and risking a pregnancy, usually with their "steady boyfriend." If these "lovers" can be persuaded to come back together by appointment at the end of normal consulting hours and if they are treated seriously and responsibly and given time, they can often be dissuaded from continuing on a course that at its most basic level could involve them in a criminal charge if the girl is under sixteen years of age. This possibility is often one they have never thought of, so blinded are they by their romantic notions. The girls are usually interested too in the possible long-term effect of taking a contraceptive pill in the early teens before an ovulatory pattern has been fully established. The specter of future infertility can be powerfully persuasive. It is, after all, the more responsible of these young people who are consulting their family doctor in the first place. As a doctor, I would not consider informing their parents, even if, as a mother, I can at least understand the sincere concern of those who disagree.

Occasionally a very promiscuous girl is referred by a social worker or by the police, and it has seemed to me that avoidance of a pregnancy is the most urgent consideration in such a case. It hardly needs to be said that I am not happy about prescribing the pill for schoolgirls for medical as well as moral reasons, but I would consider it to be preferable to a disastrous pregnancy.

Long-Acting Hormonal Contraceptives

Injectable long-acting hormonal contraceptives act in similar ways to the oral contraceptive pills and have been used by over ten million women in more than 100 countries since the early 1960s; they have been studied clinically for 25 years.[6] The medical advantages are cheapness and ease of use, while the main objection for some women is the absence or irregularity of menstrual bleeding. Once the injection has been given, treatment cannot be discontinued and the patient must be told that she is unlikely to conceive for a year after administration; there is no evidence of an adverse effect on long-term fertility.

The medical risks are in fact rather less than those of the intrauterine device (IUD), but to date they have not been approved for use in the States. The ethical objections to their use would be similar to those raised against the pill.

The Condom

The contraceptive pill has been considered first, since it requires the cooperation of a doctor. Condoms are now easily obtainable across the counter and the introduction of the AIDS factor has made their acquisition less of an occasion for embarrassment. I myself was married a long time before it dawned upon me that the barber's archetypal question, "Will there be anything else, sir?" referred to condoms. Now one sees them at the check-out of many supermarkets and available in dispensing machines.

It must be said, of course, that to observe is not necessarily to approve. None of the mainstream churches condones sexual promiscuity and all urge control and self-restraint, at least outside marriage, as being most in accord with human dignity and Christian ideals. It is well to remember, however, that the Catholic church, while fully sharing these views, also has a high tradition of realistic recognition of human frailty.

The Intra-Uterine Device

The IUD, like the pill, requires medical co-operation, usually from a gynecological or family planning clinic. It acts as a foreign body in the cavity of the uterus and discourages the implantation of a possibly fertilized ovum. If, as the Catholic church teaches, the conceptus must be accorded the right of protection from the moment of fertilization, the device is doubly condemned as contraceptive and abortifacient. Most Protestant churches, including the Episcopal, do not share this view and do not, therefore, condemn the method as intrinsically evil. In my own experience the device has never been very popular, but on medical rather than on moral grounds: some users bleed heavily and irregularly; the periods may be painful; it may be extruded; pelvic infection may occur; there is a heightened risk of ectopic pregnancy; the failure rate varies with the type of device inserted, but it is for many people unacceptably high. Pelvic infection has always been a well-recognized danger, and even when these devices were more popular few gynecologists would recommend them for a woman who had not yet borne children. Certain types—which have now been withdrawn—had a woven rather than filamentous nylon thread which acted like a wick drawing infection up into the uterus and uterine tubes. There was a considerable amount of litigation on that score in the United States, initiated by women who had suffered consequent sterility.

In spite of these possible disadvantages, their cheapness and simplicity of insertion has made them popular with large numbers of women. In many Third World countries the slight medical risks are more than counterbalanced by the much greater dangers of high multiparity, self-induced abortion, and extreme poverty. One in four pregnancies ends in procured abortion and self-induced abortion is the chief cause of maternal mortality throughout the world. It must be remembered too that if a woman dies, the death rate among her existing children rises steeply. In condemning the IUD in the cause of "life," the church must accept that it may pose a much greater threat to the lives of both women and children.

Natural Family Planning

Like many family doctors, I have been prepared to teach the rhythm method or Natural Family Planning (NFP) approved by the magisterium. Temperature and cervical mucus charts have been freely available, as well as the time necessary to explain their use. They have been much in demand by women anxious to *achieve* a pregnancy, but hardly at all by those who wish to avoid one. Those who embark on what they see as responsible family planning usually seek something wholly reliable, and, further, do not see anything particularly "natural" in the daily recording of body temperature and the viscosity of the cervical mucus.

It requires a high degree of cooperation between husband and wife, and at times when the marriage is under strain, the necessity to suppress what might be a healing demonstration of affection may seriously add to the difficulties. It must be said, on the other hand, that healthy, happy, well-instructed, and well-motivated couples can be very successful avoiding pregnancy by this method.

The method has, unfortunately, been found to be of very limited use in underdeveloped countries where poor standards of literacy and hygiene, coupled with the low status of women, militate against it. The World Health Organization reports a failure rate for NFP of 8-25 percent. Sean McDonagh, reporting on eight years of teaching the method in the Philippines, found that not a single couple, even those in daily contact with a nursing sister had been able successfully to apply it.[7]

Future Prospects

Future prospects in the field of contraception include the development of contraceptive vaccines which are being designed to provide prolonged but reversible protection against pregnancy, free from harmful side effects. Work in this field is currently proceeding in Edinburgh, Scotland, at least.[8]

One of the vaccines being developed is designed to block the surface of the ovum from penetration by the spermatozoon so that fertilization is prevented. The ease with which these vaccines could be administered on a large scale could make this form of contraception particularly appropriate for addressing the urgent family planning needs of developing countries. There is a further possibility of engineering a vaccine for men which acts on the surface of the spermatozoon and disrupts its capacity for fertilization.

The methods are still in the experimental stage, but offer promise.[9] Progress depends, of course, on the use of human ova and sperm—which is itself outlawed by the Catholic church. In centers where this work is being carried out spare ova are obtained as a by-product from IVF units or from patients undergoing simple gynecological procedures such as laparoscopy, and who have given permission for an ovum to be removed at the same time.

The Doctor and the Priest

The vast majority of patients seeking contraceptive advice are, of course, married women who want to space and then limit their families. In an area where Catholics are, admittedly, in a minority, I have found no observable difference in behavior between Catholics and non-Catholics in this matter. A glance around Catholic churches up and down the country reveals pews containing families of only average size, so I cannot think that my experience is unusual.

So where, it is legitimate to ask, does the Catholic doctor stand? If it is morally wrong to use a contraceptive it must be morally wrong to prescribe or recommend one, but the Catholic church's prohibition of artificial contraception is based on an appreciation of that same natural law by which we all derive our innate moral sense. Contraception, at least within marriage, is simply not perceived as a sin by large numbers of people who have decided nonetheless to remain within the church. If, as Pope John Paul II assures us, the teaching of *Humanae Vitae* "is written by the creative hand of God in the nature of the human person," we may wonder why so many of us are unaware of it.

Any Catholic parish priest who is normally observant cannot have failed to notice that young married couples in his parish are limiting the size of their families. Still, a homily on the subject is rarely heard and it seems to be their common experience that women simply do not mention the subject. If a woman comes to confession or for help with a spiritual problem, the priest does not ask, as she rises to go, if she is on the pill. It seems that many seminarians who are well aware of the moral dogma of the church on contraception later simply put the matter aside. An outsider observing the Catholic church could be forgiven for thinking that sexual ethics was its obsession. Instead, at ground level he would find silence. The dilemma of the hierarchy may seem to many to be as unreal as the emperor's new clothes. It is plain that contraception is being practiced widely by Catholics throughout the world, whether the bishops and magisterium accept it or not. This cannot be good for the health of the church, and the evasion and dishonesty it breeds is potentially destructive.

The issue is much more than an intellectual exercise in the application of natural law and magisterial authority to married life. An obsession with calendar watching, temperature taking, and daily examination of the cervical mucus could become an anxious ritual that threaten to displace from the center those great issues of family life the church so rightly wishes to nourish: marital stability, the good relations resulting from mutual tolerance, respect, and loving kindness between parents and children. These are not easily achieved and require an input of energy that is drained by chronic anxiety. It is hard to avoid the suspicion that the Catholic church in particular may regard a certain amount of anxiety in sexual matters to be not altogether a bad thing, as a concession or "forgiveness," in Pauline language, for what might otherwise be unmitigated sexual enjoyment by married couples.

Those, on the other hand, who have made a study of marriage tend to see the sexual bonding between husband and wife as something good in itself, which will outlast the reproductive years and help innocently to sustain the mutual comfort that a man and his wife seek to find in each other.

> Given the central role of the family in society and in Christian thought, the massive increase in marital breakdown is the single most serious social evil of Western society.
>
> The pain for the couples involved is severe and the consequences for the children frequently disastrous.[10]

I share the anxiety of some, perhaps many, Catholic doctors that if the Catholic church continues to focus so predominantly and specifically on purely sexual matters, it will be in danger of losing credence and authority on the wider aspects of human relations within marriage and the family.

Chapter 4

Sterilization

There is no doubt that the advent of the contraceptive pill caused a revolution in the attitude of women toward their fertility, which for the first time had come completely under their own control. Other contraceptives had been used for hundreds of years but there had been nothing that was at the same time both reliable and esthetically acceptable. Women were eager to take the responsibility into their own hands and no longer accepted the probability of having more children than they felt they could reasonably manage.

Those who see no ethical objection to family planning within marriage almost invariably opt for a method that is primarily reliable, even in the early years when it is used for spacing only. If so, once the family is regarded as complete, only two real alternatives remain at the moment: to continue with the pill, perhaps for another twenty years, or for either the husband or wife to consider sterilization.

Those Christian churches that do not prohibit artificial contraception—almost all the Protestant churches including the Episcopal church, and the Reformed churches throughout Europe—do not prohibit surgical sterilization either. The Catholic church, as we know, condemns sterilization as "mutilation," but it may be asked if this word has any meaning in such a context, or if it has not simply been hallowed by centuries of traditional use. As a Sister of Charity recently pointed out to me in a seminar, the church, until well into the 1800s at least, sanctioned castrated boys to sing in its chapels. A good end apparently justified this much more radical mutilation.

It is the total meaning of an act that defines its morality and the Protestant churches regard it, insofar as they express a view at all, not as mutilation but as an extension of responsible family planning. All would agree that the decision to limit the number of children should be based on Christian charity, namely, some larger good of parents and family. This good need not be pressing and urgent as in the case of abject poverty or seriously threatened maternal health, but could be simply the perceived good of having only as many children as the parents consider they can rear and educate to the standard they have set for themselves. Nor need this standard be a materialistic one, although it is often regarded as such by those opposed in principle to family limitation by any artificial means.

In the Western world there has been a dramatic drop in infant mortality in the last forty years. Before this and within the author's memory, childhood deaths were fairly common from respiratory infections, rheumatic heart disease, and tuberculosis, to name only a few. The advent of penicillin and other antibiotics and the development of immunization procedures have changed the picture significantly. A child death outside the peri-natal period (when prematurity and congenital abnormality still take their toll) is now uncommon so that a decision to regard a family as complete can be taken with relative confidence.

Population Concerns

It is outside the scope of this book to consider demographic problems in any depth, but there is an increasing awareness that the world population is rising dramatically, and that this threatens to outstrip the available natural resources to sustain it. Global population grows by a remarkable one million more births than deaths every four days, but unlike other threats to human survival, such as the accumulation of greenhouse gases, population growth is better understood and can be countered more cheaply and quickly. Even so, in Bangladesh, for example, current successes in family planning are coming tragically late; before the numbers stabilize, a population equal to that of the United States will be crammed in a country the size of Wisconsin. Many international health organizations that work to alleviate poverty and hunger see the Catholic church as seriously harming their cause.

Vast numbers of people *want* smaller families. In earlier centuries and in many Third World countries now, a high birthrate was often regarded as necessary both for the continuance of the family and as an economic necessity. High birthrates in countries with high infant mortality do not always represent, however, a volitional response to personal tragedy. When a young baby dies, lactation is cut short and with it the natural period of infertility that attends it.

One bitter consequence of curtailing family planning and voluntary sterilization programs on false economic or on religious grounds has been the heavy burden of induced abortions with their huge maternal mortality in the Third World. As I mentioned earlier, when a mother dies her existing children are much more likely to die too from poor nutrition and poor hygiene. Paradoxically, those who have wailed the most about the immorality of abortion—some American Presidents among them—have cut back on resources going into family planning and have reduced funding for effective international organizations that have supplied it in the Third World.[1] The historic fact that sterilization has been imposed in China or forbidden in Romania is, of course, an indictment of totalitarian regimes, not of the procedure itself when it is freely chosen. Unfortunately the Vatican, by virtue of being a state, was able to veto even the discussion of population problems at the International Conference on the Environment in Rio de Janeiro in June 1992.

The Married Couple

To return to our brief: typically, a married couple in their thirties, children now at school, who have used the pill to space them, decide that they are very unlikely to want to have any more. The mother may want to take up part-time work, return to a professional career, or simply want to have more time to enjoy and befriend her children and husband as the family grows up. The choice, if the couple wants to be certain, lies between continuing with the pill until the menopause has been reached, or being sterilized.

A good deal of careful research has been done on the side effects of the contraceptive pill. Thrombo-embolic disease is the best known of these, not only to the medical profession but to the public at large. The risks obviously increase the longer the pill is taken and are thought to be greater in the higher age groups. Women in their forties with a grown-up family are usually those most anxious to avoid a further pregnancy and are therefore at the greatest risk. For this reason it is becoming increasingly common to seek or to offer sterilization.

The choice then remains as to which of the married partners should have the operation, which is a decision almost invariably left to them to decide. Many women see fertility as their problem and choose to have the operation themselves. It usually involves a 36-hour admission to a hospital and a general anesthetic. Through a laparoscope the uterine tubes are occluded with plastic clamps, a method now preferred by most surgeons to diathermy which occasionally injures bowel or bladder. The abdominal incision is tiny and the woman is rarely uncomfortable for more than a week. The procedure takes effect immediately.

Many husbands, in increasing numbers in my experience, feel, on the contrary, that sterilization is their responsibility and, wishing to spare their wives surgery, decide on vasectomy. This is also easily available in most areas and is usually done as an outpatient. It can be done under either local or general anesthetic depending on the patient and surgeon's choice and judgment. The technique is simple and involves dividing the *vas deferens* on both sides. Some post-operative discomfort is usual but most men require only a day off work. It takes two to three months to become effective as some viable sperm can remain in the bulbo-urethral gland. Two negative sperm counts are therefore recommended before other contraceptive measures can be safely discontinued.

One frequently mentioned drawback after sterilization of either partner is that after stopping the pill the woman's periods revert to their normal pattern and may be both heavy and painful. A woman who has been accustomed to slight and painless bleeding while on the pill sometimes finds this unacceptable and may elect to have a hysterectomy some years later if the symptoms are severe. There is no evidence that taking the pill for a number of years in any way affects the subsequent menstrual pattern, and apart from this eventuality the menopause is reached in due course in the normal way.

The operation does not effect libido in either man or woman, and while psychological problems of inadequacy are very common in infertile men, I have not seen these after voluntary sterilization.

The slight but still significant risk of a general anesthetic has to be pointed out and considered by the patient, but the usual view is that both pregnancy and the pill have inherent dangers that more than counterbalance the risk of modern anesthesia. "Peace of mind" is usually given as the overriding factor to be considered.

It is important to point out the possibility of future regret, especially to the younger age group. With as many as one in three marriages ending in divorce this factor is highly significant and must always be considered before any decisions are made. Interestingly, it is rarely regarded as important by those seeking sterilization who have, typically, been married for eight to ten years and whose children have reached school age. They are probably the most stable marital group in society since the divorce rate is highest in the first five years of marriage and peaks again after twenty when the children are grown up.

Most women take the view that they would not want to add to their family even if, or perhaps especially if, they were to lose their husbands through death or separation. Often a happily married woman will choose to have the operation herself because in the event of her death she would hope her husband would marry again.

In an area where both male and female sterilization is common practice, I have not met a person who has regretted it, though I recognize that it must occur. While reversal may be attempted in the woman or man, it is technically difficult and the operation should never be performed unless the patient understands this.

The following patient required reassurance about the permanent effect of the procedure.

A woman came to the area having been sterilized elsewhere in her early twenties at her own request after the birth of a second mentally handicapped baby. Her teenage marriage had subsequently broken down and she had the custody of the children. In her thirties she wished to remarry and came to see me, not to ask if an attempt might be made to reverse her sterilization but to be re-assured that it "would still work." A genetic abnormality had not been demonstrated in either her or her children, although it was quite possibly present and deriving from her first husband. Both she and her prospective husband felt able to cope with her two handicapped children but not with a third child of their own, even if it were to be born healthy. They remained happily married and the children of the first marriage were loved and well cared for.

The operation was not always so readily requested as the following cases illustrate.

An older woman came to see me many years ago, when female sterilization was uncommon, though legal in certain circumstances. It involved an abdominal incision and at least a week in the hospital. She and her husband were in their late thirties and had two teenage children with Down's Syndrome. They had had genetic counseling and had been advised that the chances of a third were one in two. The children were marvelously cared for and both parents felt that their interests would be prejudiced by the arrival of another child, even if it were to be born healthy. The mother was reluctant to take the pill in view of her age, and she also had high blood pressure which is a medical bar; prolonged anxiety about another pregnancy was threatening the happiness of the whole family. She was referred to a gynecologist who performed tubal ligation without hesitation.

An immigrant Irish Catholic woman in her mid-thirties was poor and worn out with eight children and sundry miscarriages. She looked ten years older than her actual age. After her last baby, which had to be delivered in a specialized maternity unit because of the dangers of high multiparity, she told me she was "desperate" but would not consider the pill or any other contraceptive for religious reasons. I explained NFP and how to keep charts but she found it complicated and in any case her husband, though a good-natured man, was a weekend drinker and could not be counted on to cooperate. Also the Billings method is particularly unreliable in a woman of high multiparity as the cervix is often scarred and infected, as indeed it was in this woman's case. This alters the appearance and viscosity of the cervical mucus so that the time of ovulation is more difficult to recognize. She had an idea that it was possible to get permission for sterilization if medical circumstances justified it and pleaded with me to "write to the bishop." With considerable temerity I did so and received a very kind but of course negative reply. It could not have been otherwise in the immediate aftermath, for such it was, of *Humanae Vitae*. Like many highly multiparous women, she had heavy periods and her blood examination showed her to be moderately anemic. I referred her to a gynecologist suggesting that a hysterectomy might be the best solution; he wholly agreed,

so solving her many problems all at once without trans-
gressing her religious scruples. She was delighted and tackled her other family problems with new heart.

The following case was my only instance of referring an unmarried person for sterilization.

A 25-year-old girl was engaged to be married and came with
her fiancé. She had a strong family history of Huntingdon's
Chorea, her grandmother having died of it and her father
and an aunt being severely affected.

Huntingdon's Chorea is a fearsome disease that usually
manifests itself in the mid-forties by muscular un-
coordination and uncontrollable involuntary movements.
This is usually followed by severe mental deterioration. Both
her father and aunt were in long-term psychiatric institutions. Recent advances have identified the gene, but at
the time it was known simply to be a dominant gene. This
meant the girl had a 50-50 chance of carrying it and therefore of developing the disease herself in mid-life and of passing it on to her children in the meanwhile.

She wanted to get married but took the responsible decision not to have children. The man knew that his wife
might develop the disease but was willing to take the risk
and face the consequences. Adoption societies would not
have considered them with this family history. They discussed the whole problem fully, and courageously decided
to go ahead with sterilization.

Only one of the four patients quoted above had a "religious problem," although all four were practicing Christians. The Catholic
patient was saved from the harm inflicted on her by the church's
rigid teaching only by the exercise of considerable casuistry on
the part of her doctors.

Had the patient with the Huntingdon's Chorea problem been

Catholic and followed the teaching of the church, her only real option would have been celibacy, both artificial contraception and sterilization being forbidden. In the gravity of the circumstances, natural contraceptive methods would have been an irresponsible choice because of their limited reliability.

In the last few years the actual gene for Huntingdon's Chorea can be identified in the man or woman by examination of a blood sample or buccal smear taken before childbearing is contemplated. If either is a carrier, nothing can be done at the present state of knowledge to prevent the onset of disease in their own case, but if they are very anxious to have a child they might consider *in vitro* fertilization which would enable affected embryos to be discarded and only healthy ones implanted. This solution too would be proscribed by official church teaching.

Many Christian decisions involve the cross, and the girl and her husband in the last case shouldered the burden of voluntary childlessness in a very admirable way. It would seem to many to be very hard to deny them the comfort and support of marriage.

The Mentally Disadvantaged

A very different and difficult problem attracted a great deal of attention in 1987. Permission was sought by a social services department to sterilize a mentally handicapped, epileptic girl of 17 referred to in reports as "Jeanette." Permission was granted, the judge having been satisfied that it was to be performed in the girl's best interests. It was emphasized that such authorization should be exercised only as a last resort and that neither parent nor the social services department could apply for a sterilization operation without leave of the court.[2]

Those who remember the atrocities of Nazi Germany will recoil in horror from anything that smacks of eugenics, but if that immediate response can be laid aside for a moment, it could be worthwhile to consider the circumstances of the case above.

The policy in many countries with regard to mentally disadvantaged adults who have been in an institution is to return as many of them as possible to a more normal environment within the community. This seems to be rightly motivated and humane, provided adequate funds and housing are made available. In the absence of a real family it often means living in small groups under the supervision of a house-parent or a trained team of social workers. One or two of the more able manage quite well on their own in sheltered housing. They are encouraged to live, within their limits, as full a life as possible, handling their own money and doing simple shopping.

"Jeanette" was diagnosed as having the mind of a child of about 5 years in a mature adult body. She enjoyed going out with friends and was encouraged to do so within the bounds of common sense. Groups of similarly handicapped people met, to my knowledge, for a weekly social gathering in a local tavern, mixing very successfully with members of the general community. This policy almost inevitably exposes a young mentally disadvantaged woman to the possibility of sexual abuse. It would be quite impossible to reconcile the object of making life enjoyable and normal for these people with the strict 24-hour supervision advocated by those who were most vehemently opposed to the idea of sterilization.

Even at home within a family such intense supervision may not be desirable. The 20-year-old son of a patient of mine was severely mentally impaired. He was encouraged to go to a nearby store for the daily paper. Being a sociable character, he often took his time over this, looking in on friends on his way home. He was part of the community. His mother admitted she was on edge until he was back, but she thought it right not to curtail this morning routine that gave him such pleasure. It would certainly seem to be a more generous and unselfish thing that she suffered that daily anxiety than that she should have chosen the easier option of accompanying him wherever he went. Constant supervision can be both stifling and self-defeating. Nearly all able-bodied mentally disadvantaged people take great pleasure in going out by themselves to a store or to mail a letter.

"Jeanette" lacked the understanding to give permission for any kind of operation on herself, or even medication. Had she, by great misfortune, become pregnant, the social work department responsible for her would have been almost certain to present a case on her behalf for an abortion on grounds of the probability of severe psychological damage. Such a termination would necessarily have been without her consent, and the judge took account of this at the hearing.

The object of concern in such a case is not the good of society or race, but the protection of highly vulnerable persons from a trauma they are not equipped to handle. Eugenics does not come into it.

Mental handicap itself is tragic. It is not being suggested that sterilization ever could or should become a general policy; such an idea is repulsive. There might be an occasion, however, for a particular person in a particular situation when it is the least harmful option when nothing by its very nature is ideal.

In ordinary family practice my experience of Catholic patients since the Second Vatican Council is that those who see their use of contraceptives as a private matter of conscience take the same view of sterilization: they see neither as a ban to a continuing life in the church. They respect, moreover, the right of the priest to the privacy of his own views on the matter and tend not to put him into the awkward position of having to declare his true thoughts. Nor do they embarrass him by disclosing their own opinions in his presence. Both publicly and privately, there is a discreet silence over the whole issue.

The Catholic church does not disapprove of the right of a couple to decide to limit family size. Most churches view fertility control as a Christian responsibility. The difference between the churches is how this is done, and "how" is seen by many Catholics as a question considerably distanced from the core of faith.

Like many other sincere Christian believers, Catholics do not see their physical marital union in any way as a base or selfish sex drive, and consider it unfitting that it should be subjected to metaphysical scrutiny and intrusive and detailed magisterial direction.

The "natural" method of contraception allowed by the church of Rome is to some extent approved as "natural" because it does not interfere with the marital act itself, but it may be pointed out that neither the pill nor sterilization offer any difficulty on this score. Nor does the church forbid coitus in pregnancy, during lactation, after hysterectomy, or after the menopause; yet in none of these circumstances is it open to the creation of life.

For many couples the happiest time in their sexual lives is precisely after they consider their childbearing years over and they are enjoying the mutual comfort and companionship which is equally important in married life as the procreation of children.

The need to be wary of the demonstration of affection for fear of an unwanted pregnancy can be destructive of a marriage and provide fertile ground for the seeds of resentment and misunderstanding. Marriage is already a difficult undertaking as the breakdown rate clearly indicates.

Furthermore, the morality of men and women must be seen in their social context. Abraham was not seen as a bigamist in his time. In our time, a long period of non-procreative sexual life is part of our normal marital pattern and, worldwide, may be considered to be biologically necessary. The consideration of the wisdom of this and how it can be best achieved should not be outside the sphere of influence of the church; but the church in its turn might do well to call on the wisdom of all the faithful, married and unmarried, clerical and lay to contribute their judgment and to speak with authority in those fields in which they have knowledge and experience.

Chapter 5

CHRISTIAN MARRIAGE
AND SEXUAL RELATIONSHIPS
IN HANDICAPPED PEOPLE

At the beginning of 1984 the Catholic church in England earned considerable bad publicity because of the case of a disabled ex-soldier in Derbyshire who wanted to marry his Catholic nurse. The marriage tribunal of Nottingham Diocese investigated and on learning that the man was technically impotent ruled that the marriage was not permissible. By the time the Bishop of Nottingham rescinded the decision after a public furor, the damage had been done and the couple married outside the church.

After the incident, the Social Welfare Department of the Roman Catholic church set up a committee in 1985 to "assist disabled people and their care-givers to have an informed conscience in making decisions regarding their sexuality."

The report on the case was published in March 1989 under the title "Christian Marriage and Sexual Relationships in Disabled People."[1] In its background was the International Year of the Disabled of 1981, which contributed to the movement to integrate disabled people more fully into the life of the community and the social and spiritual life of the church. Known as mainstreaming, this movement reflects the current trend to move disabled people away from hospitals and large institutions into smaller residential units and wherever possible for disabled children to grow up within their own family and at a local school.

Although it is not specifically mentioned within the report, there is implicit reference to earlier harsh rulings within the Catholic church on the requirement to provide convincing evidence of the physical ability to consummate a marriage. The church, the writers plead, should apply the utmost charity and breadth in the interpretation of canon law not only in its approach to marriage but to the other sacraments as well. The benefit of the doubt should always be given, for instance, when there is uncertainty about sufficient understanding in the case of a mentally disadvantaged person.

Unfortunately the committee's work has been defeated in any practical purpose it might have served because of the scope of its agenda. It takes very little specialized knowledge of the needs and difficulties of "disabled people" to realize that those of the mentally disadvantaged, for instance, are entirely different from those of people with a purely physical disability. Chronic mental illness is not even mentioned, although it presents a problem in marriage counseling that all parish priests can expect to encounter frequently. The disorders listed in the report as causing disability in early adult life are those that primarily affect mobility and do not present any specific problem in having a sexual relationship when the time comes. It would be a simple matter to organize social help and "parish support" for a young mother with rheumatoid arthritis, for example, compared with coping with the needs and difficulties of a woman with schizophrenia or a manic-depressive psychosis. The absence of a psychiatrist on the committee is painfully obvious throughout the report.

Most enlightened education authorities will accept physically disabled children for normal schooling often with the provision that there be a special-care assistant to help with day-to-day difficulties. In such cases the report is correct when it maintains that "with understanding, both boys and girls can appreciate that their masculinity/femininity has not been affected by their disability." I had a patient with cerebellar ataxia, loss of balance and muscular coordination, who could neither walk without assistance nor write but managed normal schooling and later married and had a child.

A boy with severe spina bifida, a defect of the spine causing neurological impairment, is barely mentioned in this context, although his sexual adjustment will be an extremely difficult matter for him and his parents. Certainly it is urged elsewhere in the report that a man with paraplegia—damage to the spinal cord causing loss of power and sensation in the lower trunk and legs— should not be presumed to be permanently impotent, but that does not go very far in helping the intelligent paraplegic teenager who knows that his sexual functioning will be gravely impaired, yet finds himself strongly attracted to a girl who may be equally attracted to him. I am not suggesting that there is in fact an "answer" to such a grievous problem, but I do fault the writers of this report for not acknowledging that such a problem exists, even though it is by no means an unusual one in medical and pastoral practice. It will call for a great deal more than "understanding" because the boy's manhood *has* been grossly affected.

No mention is made either of other difficult cases when assurance about sexual function cannot be given. Anyone who has worked in a childrens' accident unit will have seen severe mutilation or even loss of the external genitalia from serious trauma, particularly burns. Extreme degrees of congenital ectopia of the bladder are usually associated with absence of the penis; in this condition—as in paraplegia—the testes are present so sexuality is likely to be normal. Plastic surgery can often restore a reasonably acceptable appearance, but erectile tissue cannot be replaced by skin graft. Girls are less susceptible to trauma for anatomical reasons but the uterus and vagina may be congenitally absent as in some cases of Turner's Syndrome. Although both common and canon law define sexual intercourse as involving penetration, I have seen lasting and happy marriages in all the above instances, though of course without progeny. All had sexual counseling and after realistic acceptance of their limitations achieved a satisfactory sexual relationship by mutual stimulation. The word "masturbation" is purposely being avoided here.

A young woman with Turner's Syndrome who married and

adopted two children enjoyed a happy marriage and was an excellent mother.

As the report rightly states, "Relationships between the sexes are not only physical. Indeed the psychological and social aspects of relationships between men and women are more important and lasting." It is good that this has been expressed, since the Catholic church is too much inclined to detailed scrutiny of the physical aspect of the marital relationship, implanting much unnecessary guilt in the process. It is doubtful that the church would have allowed the marriages described above to take place, since canon law states that antecedent and perpetual impotence on the part of the man or of the woman by its very nature invalidates marriage. The report should be commended for reminding us that *sterility* neither forbids nor invalidates a marriage.

Genetic Disease

The problem of genetic disease is tackled quite bravely in the March 1989 bishops' letter, though of course within the confines of *Humanae Vitae*. The words "family planning" are always preceded by the word "natural," but the document points out that the decision to use it does not invalidate a marriage, even when the choice has been made "to the point of not having children." When so many handicapped people form groups to provide mutual support, it would be reasonable to expect that an increasing number of them will meet each other, so this statement is valuable in that it recognizes the existence of a moral obligation not to transmit severe inherited disorders.

Sterilization is dismissed out of hand on the traditional Catholic grounds that it is a form of mutilation. "Reversible" sterilization is rather wistfully discarded as a solution, not, surprisingly enough, on moral grounds, but for the very pragmatic reason that it cannot be guaranteed to be reversible and might be regretted if the sterilized partner wishes to remarry. Reversible sterilization has been tried by inserting little plastic plugs into the uterine tubes, but unfortunately there was a considerable failure rate and a high incidence of ectopic pregnancy. Even if these technical problems were overcome, I doubt that the magisterium of the church would be ready to accept such a contraceptive method, attractive though it is from the medical point of view. What is the pill, after all, but reversible sterilization by medication?

Under the heading of Special Problems in genetic counseling the writers have selected Huntingdon's Chorea. It is a good example, one that most doctors and priests will meet at some time in their professional careers. The authors stress the gravity of the disease and the need for expert advice "especially from the priest" since an "apparently healthy person can be a carrier."

It is to be hoped that any priest so involved will be better informed about the condition than the writers of this section. The genetic marker I mentioned in the previous chapter was identified several years ago; since the gene is a dominant one, carriers will inevitably be affected sooner or later and have a 50-50 chance of passing it on to their children in the meantime. If there is a family history of this disease and the suspecting person so desires it, the test can be done before marriage is even contemplated. Genetic counseling before marriage could be regarded as morally obligatory. Most people who carry such a seriously deleterious gene would decide not to have children, and in my experience this decision was usually based on the family history alone, even before specific chromosomal diagnosis was possible in a test.

The bishops' report recognizes the dilemma and states that "direct intervention in the processes of transmission of life is not justified....However, therapeutic means to meet the illness may have secondary effects." Since they have already (correctly) stated that the disease is as yet untreatable, it would be interesting to know what this means. The most charitable interpretation might be that obscurity of meaning was intentional, since the Catholic with a family history of this terrible disease is in a most unenviable position with both artificial contraception and sterilization forbidden.

In the section on disability and sexuality the report gives too much space and attention to the problem of masturbation.

Catholic obsession with this subject is totally incommensurate with its importance and has been responsible for much unnecessary guilt and suffering in adolescence to the point where it has harmed future mature sexual relationships. Much of the theology behind it rested on ancient biology which ascribed the whole personhood of offspring to the "seed," the female contribution being seen as providing only the fertile ground.

It is easy to see how this basic misunderstanding came to be coupled with Augustine's disgust at sexual pleasure, which he considered to be justified only by procreation. Modern biology has corrected the first misunderstanding and psychology the second; it is now recognized that masturbation is normal sexual learning behavior in children and adolescents and harmful only if excessive guilt is implanted. Mentally impaired people are in many ways perpetual children and very vulnerable to guilt; all that is usually required is to teach modesty in the matter. A mother I knew who raised two mentally handicapped sons with memorable success simply restrained one or other of them when occasionally required by saying mildly "not here, darling" in the tone she would have used to correct their table manners. Both grew up to be well integrated and acceptable members of society.

When the report writers come to consider the rights of the mentally disadvantaged to a normal sexual relationship, they find themselves again on the horns of a dilemma. They submit that a relationship could develop between these people that might lead to a marriage acceptable to the church and to society. They are no doubt aware that sufferers from Down's Syndrome, for example, may be able to make and understand marriage vows. An IQ as high as 98 has been reported in Down's sufferers and it would be hard to be more "normal" than that! The authors accept at the same time that some mentally disadvantaged people who might marry are not necessarily capable of bearing and rearing children, and implicitly if not explicitly that those are the very ones who would be least likely to understand "natural" family planning methods. Tied as they are by the strictures of the church, the authors are unable to offer any solution beyond rather pious hopes that the parish will rally round.

The pill is mentioned as being therapeutically justified in some cases when a girl with a handicap is distressed by her periods or incapable of managing them, but that it could not rightly be used as a contraceptive if a sexual relationship were to develop. Are we to understand that a girl who cannot cope with periods is therefore able to cope either with a baby or with "natural" family planning? The sympathetic tone of the report makes this unlikely, and again we are left with the impression that matters are purposely left unclear. Hard though the bishops' task has been, however, it might legitimately be asked, if all really difficult questions were to be avoided or obscured, what point was there in introducing them?

The important role of conscience in all matters is repeatedly stressed, especially in the difficult matter of contraception. Perhaps they must be forgiven for failing to be more explicit about this in the ever-present shadow of *Humanae Vitae,* but if these important matters are raised, they cannot be left simply to hang in the air. Whose conscience is implicated in the case of a mentally impaired girl who might have embarked on a sexual relationship and who is totally unequipped for either pregnancy or motherhood? In these circumstances, sterilization, like the pill, is again dismissed as being an easy substitute for close and loving supervision. The *Catholic Herald* in an editorial commending the report (7 April 1989) referred to sterilization as a "counsel of despair...resulting from the pressures of official desire to tidy away problems." The fact that until recently such people and their problems were "tidied away" by being permanently locked up in institutions has perhaps been forgotten.

Social workers and psychiatrists involved in "normalization programs" for the long-term mentally ill and mentally impaired see contraception as a very important problem if their patients are to be freed from the shackles and indignities of constant supervision, however loving. Many have been discharged from chronic long-term mental hospitals after years of in-patient treatment. They are not sexually segregated, and having visitors and going out with friends is encouraged. This way of caring for such people is in no sense an easy way out; the degree of anxiety in the care-givers is intense if one of the patients fails to turn up at the expected time. The writers of the report also seem to be well aware of the need for the parents of handicapped—and they implicitly include mentally handicapped—children to be allowed the freedom to develop their full potential as people and their maximum social skills.

The question of protection does present a real dilemma for parents. "All parents have to allow their children at times to take risks....The necessity for restraint should not be used as an excuse to prevent a child from making relationships outside the family, or from broadening their experience." What is not tackled is how this admirable principle is to be reconciled with the close supervision that would be required of a teenager with a mental impairment who is developing an interest in the opposite sex but who may simply not understand the connection between sexual activity and reproduction.

The policy the bishops follow here, as in other sections of the report, of raising questions for which no real answers are suggested, or worse, of ignoring the reality of many urgent problems altogether, almost negates the value of the whole enterprise. This is very disappointing since objectives were charitable and sound and much thought and good work went into a report that might have been of great value to the church worldwide.

Chapter 6

THE STATUS OF THE EMBRYO

While agreeing on the basic tenet of the sanctity of human life, the mainstream Christian churches vary in the degree of human right they would accord to the fertilized ovum.

The Roman Catholic church in its Declaration on Abortion in 1974 (Sacred Congregation for the Doctrine of the Faith) is unequivocal. It declared:

> ...that it is not for the biological sciences to pass a definitive judgment on questions which are properly moral or philosophical such as that of the moment when the human person first exists or of the liceity of abortion. From the moral point of view it is clear that even if there be some doubt whether the entity conceived is already a human person, it is an objectively serious sin to expose oneself to the danger of committing murder. He who will be a human being is already a human being....neither divine law nor human reason admit the right of directly killing an innocent person.[1]

It is to be noted that the church does not claim in this statement that there *is* a human person from the time of conception, but that it does not know, the matter being intrinsically unknowable. Attempts have been made over the centuries in the fields of philosophy, theology, and medicine to define this time of animation but with different conclusions.

Aristotle placed the "forming and animation" of the male embryo at about 42 days and the female at about 90 days, possibly mistaking the caudal fold for the male genitalia.

Augustine drew a distinction between the formed fetus already endowed with an immortal soul, and a tissue or living entity on the way to becoming a human person.

> If what is brought forth is unformed but at this stage some sort of living shapeless thing, then the law of homicide would not apply, for it could not be said that there was a living soul in that body, for it lacks all sense, if it be such that is not yet formed and therefore not yet endowed with its senses.[2]

Thomas Aquinas, developing Aristotle's thought, clearly distinguished between the unanimated and animated fetus. "In the natural way of generation the progression is from the imperfect to the perfect. Hence in the generation of man first comes a living thing, then the animal and finally man."[3]

In the seventh century, the Penitential of Theodore decreed that a woman having an abortion after the 40th day from conception should do penance as for the more serious act of murder,[4] but in 1588 Pope Sixtus V decreed that all penalties of canon and secular law be applied to all those committing abortion whatever the age of the fetus, absolution from excommunication being reserved for the Holy See.

Since this decree met with strong opposition from moralists and theologians, Gregory XIV reverted to earlier laws and the abortion of a fetus as yet "unensouled" or "unanimated" was no longer to fall under the sanctions applying to murder.[5]

Thus matters stood in the Catholic church until 1869 when Pius IX in the declaration *Apostolicae Sedis* pronounced excommunication for all who procured abortion, without distinction as to the method or to the gestational age of the fetus, whether it were formed or unformed.

In the Episcopal church of England in 1965 a report on the subject was prepared for its assembly and was welcomed by that body, though without an official statement.[6] It pointed out that the Roman Catholic church had not always regarded the killing of a fetus before animation as murder and, while agreeing that abortion was, in the mainstream Christian tradition, undesirable, the assembly rejected the moral absolute that from the moment of conception onward a fertilized ovum had the rights of a human person.[7]

In January 1988, Dr. John Habgood, Anglican Archbishop of York, England, stated in a debate in the House of Lords that "uncertainty [regarding status] is not resolved until the cells, instead of just going through the process of multiplying as happens in the very early stages, begin differentiating." I have not heard of any widespread dissention from this view from within the Episcopal church.

In 1966 the Social and Moral Welfare Report to the General Assembly of the Church of Scotland took the view that while it regarded abortion as a serious matter, the paramount concern in the Reformed churches had traditionally been for the mother.[8]

There is thus in the Christian churches a divergence of view on the fundamental significance of the time of conception, and of the status of the human embryo. The Episcopal and Reformed churches accept the possibility of a higher right and greater good, and suggest that the intention of the moral tradition that all Christian churches share is primarily to uphold the value of human life. They consider that this intention could actually be frustrated by its narrow application in certain circumstances.

One justification that has been mentioned in support of the instant formation of a human being at the moment of fertilization is that afterward nothing particularly dramatic happens. The author of such a comment can never have been present at the birth of a live child. Once a baby has breathed, color and vigor flood the limp form in one's hands. The eyes open, the response of baby to mother and mother to baby is established in an entirely new way, and signs of individuality and personality are quickly manifest. In many years of obstetric practice I have never gotten over the drama and wonder of this moment.

It is of historical interest that in some hunter-gatherer societies that had to limit the numbers of their young for survival, the elder of the family would gently place his fingers in the nostrils of the newly born baby and it was considered that such a child had never been. It is significant that in so many languages, including Latin and English, the words used for breath, life, and spirit are interchangeable. "Inspiration" may equally signify the first breath of a newborn baby or the birth of an idea in the mind.

Roman Catholic moral teaching traditionally relies on reason as well as authority, and it is to some extent reasonable to claim that the back-dating of personhood from the time of animation to the "moment of conception" is supported by contemporary biological and genetic studies. It has been demonstrated, for instance, that all the physical characteristics of a person are genetically determined at this time. These include not only gender and other physical properties such as stature and eye color, but it seems likely that general personality tendencies are also determined at this time and in this way. Studies on identical twins who have been separately adopted and reared in different environments show that in adult life they resemble each other more closely in temperament, basic intelligence, and even artistic ability than siblings raised in the same family. A statistical resemblance has been reported even in their voting patterns and in attitudes to such matters as capital punishment, while more and more evidence is accumulating that disease tendencies in later life are also largely genetically determined. There is *some* truth in the limerick:

> There was a young fellow said damn,
> I've suddenly seen that I am
> A being who moves
> In predestinate grooves.
> I'm not even a bus, I'm a tram.

Those who find it hard to believe that a human ensouled individual is instantly formed at conception may point out that a fertilized ovum may go on to develop into identical twins. Others defend their opposite belief by suggesting that twinning may well be genetically determined and that from the beginning two persons have been present, so to speak, in the mind of God. The remerging of a twinning zygote into one has been observed in the laboratory in some mammalian species, although it has not to my knowledge been recorded in the human.

Catholic moral reasoning was largely wrought by Thomas Aquinas out of Aristotle; while there can be no doubt that biologically speaking there is from fertilization a dynamic cluster of cells with the *potential* to become a human being, to say that this *is* a human being would be to deny the whole Aristotelian concept of *hylomorphism:* the essential coexistence of material and form. Aquinas drew the moral conclusion that while deliberate destruction of a pre-animated fetus was *sinful* in that, like contraception, it frustrated the purpose of human intercourse, it could not be equated with *murder* until the fetus was animated.

If the case for human status rests essentially on "potential," it must be asked if the argument will bear the weight put upon it. The acorn, given favorable circumstances, has the potential to become the oak, but it can no more be said to *be* the oak tree than the clay on the potter's wheel can be equated with the particular pot.[9]

Fertilization is not, moreover, a "moment" but a *process* that can take up to 72 hours. In the course of maturation the sperm and ova have undergone the particular type of cell division called meiosis whereby they halve the number of their chromosomes from 46 to 23 after random exchange of their genetic material. By this means the actual combination of genes carried by each gamete is different from the next and from the parent. The uniqueness of the zygote is therefore a link in a chain of uniqueness extending back through the generations of the human species.

After penetration of the ovum, the pro-nuclei from sperm and ovum have to merge and their chromosomes to align in pairs before the pattern of the human cell nucleus is established. There is evidence that this process may go wrong as often as three times out of four, resulting in a conceptus incapable of developing into a human being. Ova that are occasionally penetrated by more than one spermatazoon are not viable nor are those with more or fewer than 46 paired chromosomes. A defective female pronucleus may lead to the formation of a hydatidiform mole, a condition known from antiquity. It consists of placenta-like cells of which all 46 chromosomes are derived from the father so that although it results from fertilization it can in no way be regarded as human tissue. If retained, it can even undergo malignant change—chorion epithelioma—and women who have had a mole have to be carefully followed up for this reason.

If merging is successfully accomplished, the resulting zygote divides rapidly, the first three divisions producing eight identical daughter cells which are themselves "totipotent," that is, they each have the ability, given the right conditions, to produce an identical embryo. If "potential" is crucial to determining status we may be forced to postulate that we have here eight potential human persons, which seems to me to be absurd.

Division occurs with increasing rapidity after this stage, with the cells becoming successively smaller. The conceptus does not gain in mass until it acquires a source of nutrition by implanting in the endometrial lining of the uterus between the fifth and seventh days. By 14 days the cells are visibly differentiating into those that will form the embryo—the "primitive streak"—and those that will form the membranes and placenta. Until the primitive streak is formed there is, strictly speaking, *no embryo*, so the term "pre-embryo" preferred by many workers in the field rests on firm biological foundations. If ovulation has occurred at the mid-point of an average 28-day cycle, it is at this 14-day stage that possibly more than half are lost in the ensuing menstrual period. The woman in this case would never have known that she had conceived. These naturally aborted conceptuses will include the ones that have failed to develop, together with those that have failed to implant.

Rarely, two primitive streaks may be formed, which may still give rise to identical twins. Conjoined "Siamese" twins result if the streaks are not completely separated; if, as the church maintains, the conclusions of science provide a valuable indication for discerning by the use of reason a personal presence from the moment of conception, the question arises as to how many persons we have here. The question cannot be side-stepped by referring to the rarity of the condition; if the ascription of an individual soul to the early embryo leads to insoluble difficulties, then perhaps the ascription needs to be reconsidered.

Many hazards still lie ahead, however, before it can be said that biological stability and secure conditions for development have been established. For example, spontaneous recurrent abortion is a major cause of infertility occurring most often between the 4th and 10th week of development, that is, between the 6th and 12th weeks of pregnancy. Some embryos implant in the uterine tube where development beyond 8-12 weeks is virtually impossible, and a much more likely outcome is rupture of the tube with death of the embryo and internal hemorrhage in the mother; some will go on to develop an abnormality so gross as to be wholly incompatible with life after birth if not aborted spontaneously earlier in pregnancy. When one considers such uncertainties it seems illogical to ascribe actual personhood to the embryo from the beginning, although highly emotive terms such as "newly conceived human being" or "unborn child" are used by those who are passionately opposed to abortion or embryo experimentation at any stage. This is eminently understandable, since the subject is intrinsically very emotive.

In one of my own pregnancies I had a threatened spontaneous abortion at 10 weeks. The bleeding settled and the pregnancy continued, but had it not, we should have gone on hopefully to start another. In that case the child I would have had would not have been the one I did have, a different "person," one might say in truth, yet in no way could a comparison have been made between the one and the other. Personhood in this sense is something that develops only after the child has developed personality.

In Edward Albee's play *Who's Afraid of Virginia Woolf?* the opposite occurs. Their son, who literally never was, is a powerful "person" in the lives of his embattled parents, but we know they are playing a game. He is a ghost without flesh and bones.

It is my experience as a doctor that in the event of an early spontaneous abortion personhood does not come to mind at all, either in mine or the patient's, when examining the conceptus which is usually presented to the doctor on a sanitary napkin. If confirmation is required, the specimen is sent to the laboratory without the need being felt for any special container or label; it is otherwise flushed down the lavatory or burned, and the patient, however distressed by her loss, does not seem to find this inappropriate. She mourns a child who might have been but never was. The church forbids baptism unless some human form can be discerned, which is clearly a highly significant difference between its theory and practice.

Without for a moment denying the unique place of the human in the order of creation, it is clear, in a post-Darwinian era, that we share much of our basic physiology with the rest of nature. Natural selection has progressed by a process of genetic variability and reproductive superabundance. All species from simple plants and animals to mammals produce more potential offspring than could possibly survive. If every sparrow's egg produced a sparrow, all other species would soon be crowded off the face of Earth.

If every fertilized human ovum were uniquely destined by God to be a person in the full sense of the word, it is hard to comprehend why so many should simply fail to develop or implant, why another should develop into an anencephalic fetus for which no personal activity can be possible, and yet another into a tumor. The latter is fairly rare, but anencephaly is among the more common causes of stillbirth. All, to my mind, are significant in that they occur at all.

We cannot, of course, know the mind of God, but neither should we be ready to ascribe to God's direct and particular will something that appears to have neither point nor reason. In addition, it seems curiously materialistic to place so much of the argument for personhood on the mere existence of a genetic structure, whether or not it goes wrong. A person is certainly more than the sum of her parts. The role of DNA in the genetic mechanism is a description, not an explanation, of God's creation of living things.

The development of a person from the ground material of her molecules may be compared reasonably to the evolution of the species. From the biochemical soup there evolved over the millennia a creature with awareness and eventually self-awareness. Teilhard de Chardin saw this self-awareness as the basis of the power of reflective thinking and the precondition for the development of the human: a being who "not only knows but knows that he knows."[10]

The human race together with fossils in rocks *could* have been created by an all-powerful God overnight, but few believe this was the way it happened. Does it detract from our image of God to postulate that the acquisition of individual personhood is a similarly continuous and gradual process and that it occurs as the embryo goes on to acquire awareness and the physical framework necessary to sustain it, in particular a central nervous system? It has been suggested tentatively by Häring and others[11] that this stage of development might be demonstrated in the fetus by the first sign of brain-cell activity that can be detected by electroencephalogram. This would fit in neatly with the current definition of death, that is, the beginning of personhood could be demonstrated by the first sign of cortical activity and its cessation by the last. It would also correct the anomaly that the church will allow doctors to define and act upon their assessment of the end of human life but not of its beginning.

A practical difficulty inherent in the suggestion is that improvement in the technique and sensitivity of electroencephalography might allow the detection of primitive embryonic cortical activity at an increasingly early stage of development; this would make the "time of animation" dependent on the sophistication of the device used to demonstrate it, which is clearly unacceptable. It would seem to be more reasonable to regard the acquisition of personhood as a seamless process that depends not only on the presence of cortical cells, but on sufficient cellular organization to support self-awareness. The withdrawal of a limb from painful stimuli, which can be observed in the early fetus or deeply comatose patient, is a function of the spinal cord and hindbrain. Not until there is a functioning cerebrum is there a capability to form relationships beyond this purely reflex response.

Being bodily present is our way of being present to the world and it is through our bodies that we communicate. Can we be bodily present before we are bodily formed?

> The body is the source of all communication....the human body is human because it is the source of human communication.[12]

> It is only by directing itself outwards toward other persons and the world that the human interiority is able to become fully a person.[13]

One thing is clear. All arguments for or against the legitimacy in certain circumstances of termination of pregnancy, embryo experimentation, and new techniques to help the infertile such as *in vitro* fertilization depend basically on the status accorded to the embryo. Some of these questions will be considered in succeeding chapters.

Chapter 7

ABORTION

One thing all Christian churches seem to agree on is that abortion is a serious matter. Roman Catholic apologists are sometimes guilty of bracketing abortion with contraception as though they were in the same ethical category, but although both are concerned with the wider issue of family limitation, it is one thing to prevent a pregnancy and entirely another to stop it once it is established. This is a conceptual difference of fundamental importance that most people recognize instantly and instinctively. Many women who will use a contraceptive without a qualm will not even consider abortion if the method fails them.

While many people may regret the easy availability of contraceptives to the young and to the unmarried, a political move seriously to restrict their availability would be unthinkable in contemporary Western society. In the UK there have been, on the other hand, several parliamentary attempts to amend the Abortion Act of 1967, all with a considerable amount of support from the public. In 1987, for example, David Alton, a Member of Parliament, introduced a bill that attracted a huge amount of attention in the media; it was directed to establishing the upper time-limit for termination at 18 weeks.

There is in most of us an innate respect for living things, and whatever has been argued in the previous chapter about the human status of the embryo, there is no doubt that it is alive. It is also unique. Compared to the genetic simplicity of other organisms, the human genetic pool is so immense that the chance of the recurrence of an identical pattern is remote enough to be discounted. We are talking, therefore, about the possible destruction of something that is not only alive but also the only one of its kind. Nature is, however, profligate with human embryos, most of which come to nothing.

While it is conceded that observing a natural process is a different matter from interfering with it, it has to be said that the whole business of medical science is concerned with doing this. There is no doubt that doctors are interfering with nature, with the very basis of natural selection, by keeping alive people who would otherwise die. Much of the world population growth in this century has been due to advances in the prevention of diseases such as malaria and smallpox and the near conquest of others such as tuberculosis. The administering of an antibiotic, for example, constitutes interference with the natural immune response. Even so, it is rarely suggested that treatment should be withheld for this reason.

Few gynecologists, however, no matter how liberal their views, would embark on an abortion with the same coolness with which they would remove an ovarian cyst, and most dislike carrying it out except for serious cause after the 12th week of pregnancy.

In this book the word "embryo" is used up to the 8th week of development—the 10th week of pregnancy—which is the period of basic formation, and thereafter "fetus" until maturity, which is the period of development and growth. The word "abortion" under this terminology at one time applied to the loss of an embryo, and "miscarriage" to the legal loss, whether spontaneous or induced, of a pre-viable fetus. Since termination of pregnancy has become more common and more widely discussed, the word "abortion" has come to carry undertones implying surgical interference. Many women and doctors, therefore, are using the word "miscarriage" for spontaneous loss at any stage of pregnancy, and "abortion" for active termination up to viability. Terms such as "inducing premature labor" and "stillbirth" lie in a gray area after about the 24th week of pregnancy.

Those gynecologists who are reluctant to terminate after the 12th week of pregnancy usually give the reason that the fetus is by that time established and becoming recognizably human. This accords, interestingly enough, with the teaching of the Roman Catholic church that baptism is not appropriate until human form can be discerned.

It cannot be said too often that women, even those who fight hardest to keep the law as it stands, giving them the choice to make their own decisions, do not actually *like* having an abortion. When Archbishop Weakland of Milwaukee reported on his "listening sessions" about abortion with groups of women, he said that even though very strong criticisms of the church's moral teaching were expressed he did not hear any defense of abortion as a good in itself, but as something no one should have to resort to. Most women are deeply upset by the procedure, even when they have judged their decision to be right and well founded.

In the UK, the Infant Life (Preservation) Act of 1929 attempted to distinguish between criminal and therapeutic abortion by stating that it would not be considered criminal if it was done in good faith to save the life of the mother, with the provision that a fetus of more than 28 weeks gestation would be capable of being born alive. In 1939 the law (Rex vs. Bourne) was extended to cover not only the mother's life but serious threat to her physical and mental health. Bourne, a gynecologist of impeccable standing, had performed an abortion, without any attempt at secrecy, on a 15-year-old girl who had become pregnant as a result of rape in particularly ugly circumstances. He was acquitted on the grounds that a woman's life depended on her mental as well as physical health.

The Abortion Law (Reform) Act of 1967 extended this concern to other children in the family and to their environment. Also, for the first time, it took into account the condition of the fetus itself, which could be legally aborted if there was a true likelihood that it would be seriously handicapped by physical or mental abnormalities.

It is of note that the Act is framed in the negative.[1] It is not worded to legalize, far less recommend, abortion in certain circumstances, but to remove the threat of criminal proceedings against both patient and doctor in such circumstances, and then only if it is agreed to after due consultation between two medical practitioners. While this distinction may seem casuistic to some, it could equally be seen to reflect the real aim of the reformers at the time.

Historical Background

In the generation of medical students to which I belonged, it was required that each student should personally conduct 20 home deliveries in the summer recess between the fourth and fifth years of study and produce a certificate to show that this had been done. Because time was short, many of us chose to go to a Catholic country such as Ireland for this purpose, where the birthrate was higher and home confinement the norm. One point was credited for a delivery and one-half for attending a miscarriage. Most of us were surprised to find that miscarriage was such a common event, usually of a fetus of about 14 to 16 weeks gestation, recognizably human but fitting into a small basin. It was usually all over before the medical student and nurse were called.

The mother had to be visited twice daily thereafter to watch for signs of sepsis or heavy bleeding, which were both common. It was some time before experience both in obstetrics and the ways of the world taught me that spontaneous abortion at this stage in pregnancy is quite rare and that many, if not most, of these had been self- or otherwise illegally induced by women made desperate by poverty and overcrowding. They had no doubt discovered by bitter and painful experience that in amateur hands attempts to terminate a pregnancy were more likely to be successful at this stage than in the early weeks. Subsequent hospital experience in Britain showed a similar dismal picture of frequent admissions of women with life-threatening sepsis or hemorrhage from the same cause. In the year preceding the 1967 Act, illegal abortion was the largest single cause of maternal death. Desperate women have always sought ways to end an unwanted pregnancy. Their situation has been likened to that of an animal in a trap: it will gnaw off its foot to escape. Even if the methods are crude and dangerous, women will use them if nothing else is available.

There is good reason to believe that the Act was aimed mainly at stopping this practice and ensuring that if a woman, usually married and poor, was intent on ending a pregnancy, it would be done early, without payment, under anesthesia, and in aseptic hospital conditions.

The Moral Dilemma

From the time of the Act there has been a conscience clause for doctors, either on grounds of religion or of allegiance to the Hippocratic Oath. The British Medical Association Handbook on Medical Ethics advises doctors that they can refuse to participate in a termination of pregnancy at any stage and in any capacity, but that they have at the same time a duty to assist the patient to obtain alternative medical advice or assistance, if she so wishes. Conscience does not absolve them in law from treating a woman when the continuation of her pregnancy is life-threatening.

The Roman Catholic church stands alone among the mainstream churches in Britain in condemning abortion under all circumstances. It takes its moral stand on the "safety-first principle," namely, that since what is proposed to be destroyed *could* be a person, then the risk must not be taken.

The traditional analogy of the deer in the woods is often used in moral teaching: if a deer hunter saw a movement in a bush that was *almost certainly* a deer but could just *possibly* be a man, then he should not shoot. This analogy is not altogether apt, however, because in real life it is more likely to be the difficult matter of weighing the serious claims of a woman who *most certainly* is a person against those of the embryo or pre-viable or non-viable fetus who only *might* be. The magisterium is, however, clear in its direction: all human beings are equal in the sight of God and to kill even a potential human being is against the dictates of natural law.

The Episcopal and Reformed churches are not absolute in claiming equal human right for the embryo or even the more mature fetus; they take into account what they regard as the greater rights of the mother. They also maintain that severe handicap can justify termination, though there are of course personal differences with regard to what is meant by "severe." In the Jewish and Islamic traditions the rights of the fetus are regarded as secondary to those of the mother, whether before or after animation.

Doctors and nurses who are totally opposed to abortion under any circumstances are probably wise if they avoid hospital practice in obstetrics and gynecology, but other branches of hospital medicine are not entitely problem-free in regard to cooperating in what might be immoral. An anesthetist, for instance, might have qualms about colluding indirectly in a termination. In moral theology the classic degrees of "cooperation in the sin of another" make few allowances for living in a pluralist society, and it is increasingly difficult to know where collusion begins and ends.

Some family practitioners who for religious reasons take an absolutist view on abortion, simply tell their patient they will have nothing to do with it and that they must approach someone else. This policy is eminently understandable but unsatisfactory for several reasons. First, doctors have a professional duty to help their patients obtain alternative advice, and not simply wash their hands of them. Another doctor may be known to be sympathetic to abortion, in which case there is a degree of collusion only one step removed from direct referral. It also invokes the dubious morality of asking another person to take on the burden of something that the referring doctor has rejected as intrinsically sinful. If the other doctor is known to be unsympathetic, the referring doctor is failing in his professional duty to the patient.

My own policy was to take the responsibility for referral myself. If after a full discussion with a patient I thought the grounds for abortion were trivial, I stated in the letter to the consulting gynecologist only the relevant medical information and why the patient herself thought the pregnancy should be terminated. I would tell her that it was a matter to be decided between her and the surgeon who would actually do the operation. This ultimately applies, of course, in all hospital referrals, gynecological and otherwise. In an area where family planning advice was readily available and known to be so, or, even more significantly in an area with a stable populace comparatively free from inner-city anonymity, the situation described here was quite rare.

It is difficult to justify imposing one's moral teaching on others, especially those who have well considered moral values of their own.

Catholic doctors should be wary, then, of judging their professional colleagues who may not share the stricter view of the Roman Catholic church. It must certainly not be assumed that they ignore the ethical dimension. Most, in my experience, give such matters deep thought, even though they may come to a different conclusion.

Since the British Infant Life (Preservation) Act was framed in 1929 and amended 10 years later, life-threatening complications in the mother have become much less common. Nephritis and rheumatic heart disease, for example, were both caused by the prevalence of infection with the hemolytic streptococcus, which has since been conquered by a combination of better housing and penicillin. Nevertheless, I remember some life-endangering conditions of a few patients whose pregnancies were legally terminated before the Abortion Act of 1967. One was a severe diabetic with renal complications whose only previous pregnancy had caused her diabetes to escape control in spite of careful in-patient monitoring, bringing both her and the baby close to death. She was advised never to risk another pregnancy. Today she would be offered sterilization after delivery. Another was a mature unmarried woman whose discovery of her pregnancy after a single sexual lapse was followed by a near-successful suicide attempt and who would almost certainly have attempted another if the pregnancy had been allowed to continue.

Because so many people seem to think of termination of pregnancy as the exclusive concern of young, irresponsible unmarried girls, I quote the following case in some detail:

A man I knew well had an appointment one evening. He was a quiet, respected member of the community with a large grown-up family who had all done credit to their good upbringing. The youngest was about 20, and they had several grandchildren. He was painfully ill at ease and it was several minutes before he could bring himself to say what the problem was. His wife, whom I also knew well, was 47 and when she missed a period she had put it down at first to the beginning of menopause. Her last pregnancy at age 39 had ended in an alarming spontaneous abortion at about 10 weeks, requiring emergency blood transfusion and transfer to a hospital by the medical emergency squad. Since then they had been "very careful" in their marital relations, and she had had a repair of prolapse with amputation of the cervix. This operation predisposes to miscarriage should a further pregnancy occur and is rarely done now, most surgeons preferring vaginal hysterectomy. She had soon realized, from previous experience, that she was in fact pregnant and had secretly sent off a urine specimen for testing. This had confirmed her fears. She was now at about the ninth week and, since her discovery, had become alarmingly withdrawn, neither speaking nor leaving the house. She had never wanted to have anything to do with abortion or considered that the issue would ever touch their lives. It was with the greatest reluctance that her husband finally managed to ask if I thought they might be helped under the terms of the new Act. He was deeply, though quite unjustifiably, ashamed that it had happened at all, and even more that he should even be thinking of this way out. He brought his wife the following morning and I referred her at once to a gynecologist for his opinion. He considered that she had strong grounds for termination on account of serious threat to both her physical and mental health. He was also convinced that her chances of carrying the pregnancy to term were in any case negligible and had charitably conveyed this conviction to her and her husband. As a result, I do not think that either of them suffered from significant guilt problems from having the abortion. She was sterilized during the same admission.

The Roman Catholic church holds as moral the removal of an embryo or fetus as a side effect of an operation, the direct intent of which is to remove a diseased organ and save the patient's life. The example usually given is that of a cancerous uterus when the objective is a timely hysterectomy, and only incidentally termination of the pregnancy, which is undesired but also unavoidable. This is the principle of double effect.

Many thoughtful Christian people including those of the Episcopal and the Reformed churches do not see a significant moral difference between this situation and the removal of a fetus in other life-threatening conditions, such as kidney failure or severe hypertension. They might see the objective, as in the first case, to be the saving of maternal life and the sacrifice of the fetus as the only means of achieving it. They hold that the principle of double effect is equally applicable in those other cases.

In the first case, according to the Catholic position, the death of the fetus is an unintended result of the operation, but in the other cases the killing of the fetus, which will save the mother's life, is directly intended as a means to that end. It is immoral, the argument goes, even in a case like this, to directly pursue evil means (killing the fetus) to achieve a good result (saving the mother's life).

Ectopic Pregnancy

Pregnancy in a cancerous uterus is rare, but the condition of ectopic pregnancy is common. The Roman Catholic church allows removal of the uterine tube together with embryo in such circumstances, viewing it in the same light as the cancerous uterus. This is a less straightforward case, however, for the strict application of the absolute ethic. The uterine tube is a "diseased organ" only in the sense that it contains an embryo that is distending it. Almost always if left alone it will rupture and cause serious hemorrhage in the mother. The diagnosis is usually made before this catastrophe occurs and the tube together with embryo is removed prophylactically. Cases have been reported, however, of the diagnosis having been missed and of the pregnancy continuing in the abdominal cavity with the placenta attaching itself to internal organs. A live baby has been delivered at term by caesarean section, after this abdominal pregnancy. It is certainly a rarity but one we were taught as students to keep in mind. I have seen one case of it.

An immigrant worker who had had no prenatal care knew she was pregnant and that her time was about due. She arrived at the maternity hospital, in labor. She was a thin woman and on abdominal examination the fetal parts seemed to be extremely well defined as though they were just under the skin. Sometimes multiparous women have a very thin uterine wall and this seemed to be the likeliest explanation, but she told me that it was in fact only her second pregnancy. The fetal heart was heard very clearly. There was a great deal of fetal movement and the head was still high above the pelvic brim. She was vague about the history of the early months of her pregnancy but had never had pain severe enough to consult a doctor. I referred her at once to a major obstetric hospital where she was delivered abdominally of a full-term healthy baby, which had developed outside the uterus. The placenta had attached itself to her bowel and bladder, and since surgical dissection would have been impossible it was left behind. At her postnatal examination she was perfectly well and the placenta appeared to have been largely absorbed.

I have never personally seen another case, though one was reported in September 1988, but it must occur from time to time in less developed countries where prenatal care is sketchy and medical attention in the early months of pregnancy is not always available or even sought.

Could there be a moral case, therefore, for leaving an ectopic pregnancy alone on the slight chance that it might be that very occasional one that survives? If the 6-8-week embryo really has equal rights as the mother, the answer would have to be yes. It would certainly develop at grave risk to maternal safety, but so does the one whose mother is in renal failure.

Once again it would seem that attempts to apply absolute rules to particular cases lead not only to impossible medical dilemmas but to philosophic and theological muddles.

Fetal Screening for Neural Lesions

In prenatal care it is routine practice to measure the level of alpha-feto-protein in the maternal blood at the 17th week. Blood can be taken at 15-16 weeks but is less reliable and a doubtful report would have to be repeated. This blood test reflects the level of the alpha-feto-protein in the amniotic fluid surrounding the fetus, and a high reading suggests the presence either of twins or of incomplete closure of the neural tube that encloses the spinal cord, loosely termed spina bifida. Further serial readings will indicate whether the defect is tending to close or to remain open. Ultrasound screening, if it has not already been done, will distinguish twins from a neural tube defect.

Anencephaly

By 12 weeks ultrasound will reliably diagnose anencephaly, which is spina bifida in its severest form. In this condition the parietal skull and most of the cortex is absent; only the lower brain that controls basic bodily functions is present. On delivery a few gasping breaths may be taken but the condition is incompatible with life. Such an incomplete fetus has commonly been regarded as discarded biological material and if the mother has given consent, it may be used as a valuable tissue source for teaching or research purposes. At the present state of the law in most countries it cannot be used for organ donation, an anomaly that will be discussed later (Transplant Surgery).

Anencephaly, together with the less severe spinal neural defects, has a genetic element. A woman who has had one affected child has an increased risk of having another, the chance of a second being on the order of one in twenty, and of a third (having had two) of one in eight. A higher risk of complications of pregnancy is associated with congenital fetal abnormalities, particularly hydramnios, antepartum hemorrhage, and pre-eclamptic toxemia. In anencephaly, therefore, the woman is carrying at increased risk to herself a baby who will not survive birth.

The Roman Catholic document of 1987, "Is Prenatal Diagnosis Morally Licit?" condemns termination in all circumstances; x-rays are vaguely mentioned, a term that presumably refers to ultrasound screening.[2]

In the case of anencephaly, to induce premature labor in order to terminate the pregnancy is analogous to turning off the life-support system in a "brain-dead" person, the system in this case being the maternal placental circulation. There must be a few doctors who would hesitate to initiate this, knowing that the mother bears not only an increased physical risk, but the psychological agony of carrying a child who will not survive.

The following patient was particularly unfortunate.

A woman after a normal pregnancy without hydramnios or any other warning sign was delivered at term of a baby with gross spina bifida, the whole length of the spinal cord being exposed. It breathed only intermittently and was placed in a cot where it died after about half an hour. About 2 years later, before the screening techniques mentioned above were available, she had a second pregnancy. This time she developed hydramnios at about the 30th week and because the x-ray showed an anencephalic fetus, premature labor was induced. A few years later screening became available for such high risk cases. This involved amniocentesis at about the 16th week. With the promise that this would be done, she felt she could risk another pregnancy and this time happily had a normal baby. She decided not to risk having any more and was sterilized.

Spinal Neural Defects

This term, which is medically preferred to "spina bifida," covers the whole range of conditions arising from failure of the neural tube to close; the severity varies from the whole length of the spinal cord being exposed to a small mid-line defect of the sacrum, which may be found accidentally on x-ray examination later in life. The possibility is uncovered by the blood test done at the 17th week of pregnancy, and corroborative amniocentesis is indicated today only if the level of alpha-feto-protein is raised in the maternal blood. While anencephaly can be confidently diagnosed before 12 weeks, it is not until about 17 weeks that less gross spinal neural defects can be picked up by ultrasound screening. Some of these are not necessarily incompatible with life, but accurate surgical and neurological assessment is not really possible until after birth. If the defect is limited to the lower spine, skin coverage is often successful and, though the person is likely to be paraplegic, they may lead a rewarding and happy life. Those with a surgically treatable lesion are, however, in a minority and the outlook for spinal neural defect is generally bleak.

Non-Neural Abnormalities

Non-neural abnormalities, such as congenital absence of both kidneys and the grosser cardio-pulmonary defects, can also be picked up by ultrasound screening in expert hands. These are compatible with life only if immediate transplant surgery is available. This possibility is remote, though, and most people would doubt even its wisdom. The reaction of many viewers to the nightly pictures on television news a few years ago of a tiny baby who survived 10 days after heart transplant was that she might well have been better left to die in peace.

In the case of a baby who will inevitably be stillborn, there seems, to my mind, to be little in the way of a moral problem for either doctor or patient in cutting short the pregnancy. For those conditions that are not mortal but very seriously life-threatening, both parents and obstetricians are faced with a very difficult decision about what action, if any, should be taken. Some patients, by no means all of them Catholic, prefer to avoid the possibility of such an agonizing dilemma and simply reject the initial blood test, preferring not to know.

It is a known fact, however, that congenital abnormality and prematurity—often associated—are now the main causes of neonatal mortality, and the benefits of this screening program are widely accepted by most of the medical profession and by the public at large. Unfortunately, even with perfect patient compliance—no missed appointments—perfect and speedy communication between laboratory and family doctor, and instant admission to a specialist unit for amniocentesis, it is very difficult before 18 to 20 weeks to assemble the information, discuss the findings with the patient, and allow her time to consider them before deciding what action, if any, shall be taken.

Prenatal Screening by Amniocentesis

Amniocentesis consists of passing a fine needle through the mother's abdominal and uterine walls into the amniotic cavity surrounding the fetus in order to remove a few millilitres of fluid for laboratory examination. It is technically difficult before 15 to 16 weeks to obtain adequate amounts of fluid for testing. Biochemical estimate of alpha-feto-protein was discussed earlier when it is used to corroborate raised maternal blood levels. Other biochemical tests can reveal the onset of rhesus problems and some rare diseases of defective metabolism. The detection of the latter, however, may require laboratory incubation for 6 weeks or more, by which time the fetus might be viable. Additionally, cells are shed from the fetal and placental tissues into the amniotic fluid and these can be examined for chromosomal abnormalities, with laboratory results in 10 to 20 days.

Amniocentesis is fairly simple but not entirely without problems: slight bleeding might occur which, while in itself not serious, would invalidate laboratory findings because of contamination of the specimen. In a small but significant number of cases (0.5 - 1 percent) it can precipitate a miscarriage. There is a practical problem in that although obtaining the specimen may take only a few minutes, the laboratory examination is time-consuming and expensive and available only in specialized centers.

For these reasons amniocentesis is not regarded as a routine screening measure. The results would not justify the risk or the extravagant use of laboratory time. It is reserved, therefore, for those cases where there is a heightened risk of abnormality, the best known of these being Down's Syndrome, which is more common in babies born to women in the older age group, whether or not she has previously had normal children. There is a demonstrable chromosomal abnormality in Down's, but it is not clear why it should manifest itself more commonly in the children of older women.

If a young woman gives birth to a child with Down's Syndrome, it is customary to examine the mother's body cells for chromosomal abnormality. These cells can be obtained from a blood sample or from a smear taken from the inner side of the lip, a "buccal smear." If she is found to be a genetic carrier of the condition, the chance of a further affected child is one in two. Such women and those over the age of 35 are offered amniocentesis. It should be noted that while all Down's children share a similar chromosomal abnormality, some can be more severely handicapped than others. Some will have additional somatic abnormalities such as a congenital heart lesion or intestinal blockage.

A test was developed in 1992 that promises to detect Down's Syndrome by means of a simple blood examination that can be carried out at the same time as the alpha-feto-proteins are measured at the 17th week of pregnancy. A positive result would have to be confirmed by amniocentesis, but the present indications are that it promises to be both accurate and inexpensive.

Whether or not Down's Syndrome constitutes grounds for termination is regarded by most gynecologists as one of the most difficult of all decisions and essentially a matter for the woman herself to decide. Most of them would offer termination before fetal viability if the patient so wished it, on the grounds, under the British 1967 Abortion Act, of serious mental handicap. My advice to those many women who would find such a decision impossible is to decline the test. Many women do so, and most have already decided on this for themselves earlier in pregnancy, as the following case illustrates.

A patient was dismayed to find herself pregnant at the age of 44, but had not even considered abortion. She and her husband had four teenage children, one of whom was physically and mentally disabled with cerebral palsy. This child lived at home but attended a Day Care Center for severely impaired children. The other three were healthy. The mother felt able to cope with another baby, but fervently hoped it would be "all right." They were not a Catholic family. Although she was eligible, she declined amniocentesis for screening for Down's Syndrome. At about 26 weeks she developed slight hydramnios and was referred to the consulting obstetrician who agreed on this finding. Over the next two weeks the amount of fluid increased markedly and she was admitted to the hospital for therapeutic amniocentesis to relieve intra-abdominal pressure. Alpha-feto-proteins were normal and it was several weeks before chromosomal analysis came through by which time she was 31 weeks pregnant. There was a chromosomal abnormality of Trisomy

18 pattern, known as Edward's Syndrome. This is associated with multiple gross abnormalities and, in the rare event of the baby surviving birth, it is virtually inconsistent with life beyond immediate infancy. In this case, ultrasound demonstrated the gross cardiac abnormalities and underdeveloped lungs that are common in such infants, and the patient was offered and accepted termination on the certain prediction of a stillbirth or neo-natal death. It was in fact a stillbirth, and post-mortem examination showed, as well as other multiple somatic abnormalities of kidneys, bladder, digestive tract, and limbs, the cerebral malformation and cortical cell abnormalities that are the essential features of this syndrome, and render meaningful life impossible.

Fetal sex is also revealed in the process of chromosomal examination, but the only medical indication for specific sex determination would be the presence in the family history of severe sex-linked congenital disease, such as some of the muscular dystrophies.

No doubt the number of serious chromosomally recognizable conditions such as Edward's Syndrome will increase with advances in the field of genetics. It must be said that it is both unfair and unfounded to regard professional research workers in this field as being even marginally concerned with breeding a super-race or "designer babies," although this charge is often levied.

The diagnosis and termination of pregnancy for such relatively minor conditions as club foot and cleft lip are frequently mentioned by anti-abortion campaigners, but have no basis in medical practice. After extensive inquiry I have not found a single ultrasound specialist who would claim to be able to diagnose either of these conditions prenatally, nor an obstetrician who would consider terminating a pregnancy on their account.

Termination on grounds of sex alone will be considered later.

Screening and the David Alton Bill

In 1987 the public debate in the aftermath of David Alton's Private Member's Bill to reduce the upper time limit for abortion to 18 weeks demonstrated vividly the difficulty of framing legislation for an issue as highly emotive as abortion. In the media and in the legislature the protagonists tended to present their cases as sincere but irreconcilable convictions. The politicians, in so far as they contributed to the debate at all, tended to split along party lines.

The legal maximum of 28 weeks was not in fact contained in the Abortion Act, but was a remnant of the Infant Life (Preservation) Act of 1929. The Alton Bill might well have had a much greater chance of acceptance had it not been so specific. Eighteen weeks was an unfortunate choice from the screening point of view, for reasons given earlier, and failed to win the support both of the medical profession at large, and of important medical organizations.

It can be argued, furthermore, that a fetus of 18 weeks looks and behaves much as it does at 17 or 19 weeks. No particularly dramatic development takes place at this point; the organs are complete long before this date, but it is not until nearer 24 weeks that the lungs are able to function usefully. Even at this stage there is a lack of tension-lowering substance (surfactant) in the alveolar air spaces, which is necessary for inflation and oxygen exchange. Although survivals at an even lower degree of prematurity are recorded, they are exceptional even in a highly sophisticated premature unit. For this reason, the judge in a much publicized court case in England in 1987 found that a fetus of less than 24 weeks was "incapable of being born alive."[3]

The legal definition of a live birth is now tending to be directed to function of the lungs rather than of the heart and other visceral organs.[4] It should be noted that "premature" relates to actual body weight at birth rather than to the gestational age, which is never more than an estimate. Neo-natal physicians have been publicly criticized in the last few years for deciding to make no attempt to resuscitate certain grossly premature infants. It would be very regrettable if various "pro-life" groups, however well intentioned, were to force neo-natal physicians to act more from fear of litigation rather than from sound clinical judgment. This seems to be the case all too often in the United States where pediatricians and obstetricians in particular can scarcely afford their insurance premiums. This is less of a problem in the UK, but even so, there was considerable relief in the profession when a Glasgow Sheriff Court in 1988 upheld the decision of a doctor not to put a grossly premature baby on a ventilator.

A proposed limit of the 12th week of pregnancy for abortions would have made more sense from the embryological point of view, and might have received more enthusiastic support from those who were reluctant to lend their weight to anything less than a complete ban on abortion. "After a viable age" would have been likely to command the wholehearted support of most of the medical profession and would have prevented at least the scandal of termination at a stage when other babies may be receiving intensive care in a premature unit; this is deeply repugnant to the medical and nursing profession as well as to the general public. The Alton proposal was defeated but the upper limit was changed from 28 to 24 weeks except in the case of severe fetal handicap. Since the occasional infant survives even greater prematurity than this, the medical preference for "after a viable age" would have been more acceptable and is in fact the criterion used by most practitioners.

Chorionic Villus Sampling

During the months before the debate on the Alton Bill there was a great deal of discussion in the media of Chorionic Villus Sampling (CVS) for the detection of chromosomal abnormalities. By this technique a tiny sample of fetal membrane or placenta is obtained by passing a fine hollow needle through the cervix of the uterus. Since the cells obtained by this means arise from the same fertilized ovum as the embryo, they have the same chromosomal pattern. It can be performed by experts in the procedure at about the 8th week and for that reason has obvious advantages over amniocentesis, which must be performed later. The benefits to the patient are both physical and psychological. If the result indicates an abnormality sufficient to justify termination, it can be done at a much earlier stage with greater technical ease, reducing the physical and mental trauma to both patient and surgeon.

Those supporters of the Alton Bill who maintained that this new procedure precluded the need for later and more established screening programs were, however, simply mistaken. Although spinal neural defects—by far the most common abnormality—undoubtedly have a genetic component, this has not so far been demonstrated. These defects cannot be detected, therefore, until the fetus has passed that stage of development when the neural groove has normally closed.

Only chromosomal abnormalities can be demonstrated by CVS, and although the number of congenital abnormalities recognizable by this means will no doubt increase, they are as yet comparatively few. The technique is more difficult than amniocentesis, and laboratory interpretation is time-consuming, highly specialized, and not yet infallible. The danger of causing accidental abortion is considerable, much higher than with amniocentesis. For these reasons it is offered only to those women who have a high risk of producing a child with serious genetic handicap. This might include a woman who has had a previous Down's infant and who herself has been shown to carry the abnormal gene. Since the risk of a second affected child is one in two, this might be considered to outweigh the risk of the procedure itself. It would not be justified as part of a screening program for an older but otherwise normal woman with previous healthy children. In obstetric units where it is offered, the test is confined to those with a family history of severe chromosomally recognizable genetic disease, or where serious hereditary disorders are sex-linked, as mentioned earlier.

With ever-increasing success rates for *in vitro* fertilization, it becomes practicable and morally more acceptable to offer embryo selection to carriers of seriously deleterious genes so that only unaffected embryos are implanted into the uterus. This has been successfully accomplished for conditions such as Duchenne's muscular dystrophy and fibrocystic disease.

Some people may consider such human scientific enterprise to be "unnatural" or "playing God," but nature may be at times seriously deficient in its structure and manifestations. Is it not equally reasonable to suggest that it is part of human nature to be intelligent and inventive and, having been made in the image of an intelligent, enterprising and loving God, that we should aspire to continue God's handiwork?

Sex Selection

Reports of requests for termination of pregnancy on grounds of sex alone have caused occasional scandal in the press. Horrifying as it may sound, a case can be argued that as much psychological damage is inflicted on women of certain ethnic communities by the repeated bearing of female children as on others who have their pregnancies legally terminated because of different threats to their psychological health. Such women may face divorce and family ostracism and have been known to suffer from suicidal despair. The opinion, in a personal communication, of one gynecologist deeply involved in professional ethics was that termination in such a case might be considered to be ethically acceptable only if very stringent conditions were met: that the marital and family pressures were sufficiently severe, that the woman had at least two previous daughters, that she accepted diagnosis by CVS, not the later and technically easier amniocentesis, and that she understood and accepted the considerable risk of accidental abortion inherent in CVS. She must also understand that such an accidental abortion, if the conceptus proved to be male, might represent her only chance of having had a male child.

Sex determination by pre-insemination selection of male and female spermatozoa is still in the experimental stage.

Post-Coital Contraception

Interceptive methods of contraception that prevent implantation are considered in this chapter since they effect their purpose after the ovum has been exposed to the possibility of fertilization and might therefore be considered as abortifacient in the strict sense of aborting a biological process of development. They include the intra-uterine device, some contraceptive pills, the "morning after" pill, and menstrual extraction. The first two were considered in the chapter on contraception.

Menstrual extraction is performed, or a drug to induce bleeding is administered, as soon as a period has been missed or in the expectation of a missed period before a definitive diagnosis of pregnancy can be made, if indeed it has occurred at all. This would seem to many people to be a preferred alternative to possible formal termination several weeks later in the case of rape, or of abuse of a sexually mature child. The laws relating to abortion refer to termination of a pregnancy or procuring a miscarriage. If a post-coital procedure is carried out before implantation has had time to occur, can there be termination of pregnancy in the absence of true pregnancy, or a miscarriage in the absence of true carriage?[5]

The magisterium of the Roman Catholic church condemns menstrual extraction, or induction of bleeding by hormones, even in the case of rape or child molestation on the ground that the fertilized ovum has the intrinsic right to implant. Many, both within and outside the church, will find this position difficult to accept, and indeed there was an instruction of the British Catholic hierarchy in 1980 stating that a raped woman is "certainly entitled to seek immediate medical assistance with a view to preventing conception."[6]

This seems to leave a loophole in the church's general prohibition of contraception, and it is dificult to know what "medical assistance" the bishops had in mind. Sperm will enter the cervical mucus within 90 seconds after ejaculation, which readily explains the poor performance of the traditional remedy of post-coital douching. In 1985, the bishops maintained that estrogens to prevent ovulation could be administered to a raped woman, provided she was in the first half of her mentrual cycle when the offense occurred. This assistance was not licit for a woman who had been unfortunate enough to be raped in the second half of her cycle when there might be the possibility of endangering the life of an unborn child.[7]

The church does not pretend, of course, that a pregnancy resulting from rape does not present an acute problem to the person raped and to society. It would urge us to rise here as in all other cases of contemplated abortion to heights of compassion and self-sacrifice worthy of human beings, using all the material and spiritual resources available to us.

The intrinsic value of such a general view is not lightly ignored. Christianity can involve the cross, but we are left with the question of compassion to whom? To a not-yet-implanted zygote, or to the victim of rape or child abuse? Could a child, especially, be asked to make or even understand this kind of self-sacrifice?

RU 486, "The Abortion Pill"

The naturally produced hormone progesterone is necessary for the continuation of a pregnancy, and RU 486 (mefepristone) acts by blocking its action. It was developed in France and is now available in several European countries, but not in the States.

Taken in tablet form and used alone within 10 days of a missed period, it will induce abortion in 85 percent of cases. It also increases sensitivity to prostaglandin and is usually reinforced by giving a small dose of this drug 48 hours later as a vaginal pessary.

It is licensed for use only until the end of the 8th week of pregnancy which is the 6th week of embryonic development. In the UK it must be administered under hospital supervision and under the terms of the Abortion Act. In case of failure and possible adverse effects on the developing embryo, it is required that the patient sign an agreement to proceed to surgical termination if the method is unsuccessful.

There is no evidence as yet to suggest that it leads to *more* abortions in countries where termination is already legal, but it should certainly make for *earlier* abortion by eliminating the need for an anesthetic and hospital admission.

In the Third World, unskilled termination of pregnancy heads the causes of maternal death, and the World Health Organization has stated that "although abortion is not acceptable as a family planning method, the WHO accepts that safe and effective medical methods of early termination of pregnancy have the potential for less adverse effects than surgical methods and is continuing research on RU 486."

In the whole field of abortion the well-worn saying that every case and every situation is different is platitudinous, but still true. We are required each time to make the notoriously difficult decision about who has the greater claim to be our neighbor.

Chapter 8

INFERTILITY

Since the birth of the first test-tube baby astounded the world in 1978, amazing advances have been made in the field of human infertility. The rapid and indeed alarming pace of development led to the establishment in the UK of a *Departmental Committee of Enquiry into Human Fertilization and Embryology,* which was chaired by Oxford philosopher Dame Mary Warnock and published the Warnock Report in 1984. Most of the recommendations of that report were adopted by the British Parliament in *The Human Fertilisation and Embryology Act of 1990.*

It is proposed here to consider in two main categories the various techniques that have been developed: those that are directed to the production of a child who would be the true genetic offspring of both its parents, namely, artificial insemination by the husband (AIH) and *in vitro* fertilization (IVF); and those that require not only technical assistance but the introduction of a third person into the equation, namely, donor insemination (DI) and surrogate motherhood (SM).

Embryo transfer—"womb leasing"—and egg donation are still largely experimental and will be considered briefly later.

AIH was the first to be tried and was condemned by Pope Pius XII on two counts: it separated procreation from the marital act, and obtaining sperm by masturbation was considered to be intrinsically immoral.

This view was not shared by the ethical advisors to the Anglican (Episcopal) church, which in their report to the Feversham Committee in 1960 withdrew their previous scruple about masturbation.

In the Roman Catholic submissions to the Warnock Committee in 1983, several Catholic bodies, including the Guild of Catholic Doctors, were prepared in general to accept AIH. They also agreed with the Anglican Commission that masturbation with the object of obtaining semen for fertilization purposes was totally different from that "directed in procuring solitary and self-centered pleasure," and recommended that a different word be used.[1]

In 1987, however, in its *Instruction in Respect of Human Life in Its Origin and the Dignity of Procreation*, the magisterium of the Catholic church condemned all the new techniques for the treatment of infertility.[2] No attempt was made to differentiate between the methods that led to a genetically true child of its parents from those that did not. A child born of AIH or IVF has a father who is the real father and a mother who is the real mother; it has parents who have a normal continuing marital relationship, and it is born after a normal pregnancy and delivery. In DI and SM, on the other hand, the child is the true genetic offspring of only one of its parents and therein lies, one would have thought, the crucial difference and nub of the moral, legal, social, and psychological problems that follow.

The central moral objection of the Congregation of the Doctrine of the Faith that led it to condemn out of hand even the so-called simple case of *in vitro* fertilization appears to have been exact locus and context of fertilization, a point I find difficult to grasp. Also its banning of "masturbation" to obtain sperm precludes not only AIH but the very diagnosis and investigation of male infertility. The suggestion was made that the church might allow the collection of semen from a condom supplied with small perforations which would circumvent the accusation of contraceptive intent, but are not inanimate objects generally understood to be morally neutral? A bread knife is not a weapon unless it is used to kill somebody. Can a condom be a contraceptive if it is used to collect semen for subsequent fertilization? If not, holes are superfluous. Such thinking threatens to invite ridicule upon the church and is painful to those of us who care about its central doctrines and public image.

Artificial Insemination by the Husband (AIH)

About one in ten married couples has a fertility problem and about half of these are due to male infertility. If the woman has a normal menstrual history and the pelvic organs seem to be healthy on clinical examination, it is customary to investigate the husband before submitting his wife to more invasive diagnostic tests.

I have had only one Catholic male patient who refused to produce a specimen of semen for examination because of the church's teaching on masturbation. A post-coital test was done but failed to show any active sperm; the test was inconclusive but there was no medical indication to subject his wife to further investigation and the case had to be closed. Sadly, they remained childless.

If there is a total absence of sperm in the semen, attempts at hormonal treatment have, unfortunately, a low success rate. If the count is merely low, AIH is usually given a trial by injecting stored and concentrated semen into the uterus at the time of ovulation.

If a low count is accompanied by low sperm mobility, their fertilizing potential may be tested *in vitro,* using prepared hamster ova. If fertilization occurs the resultant cell division is stopped at the two-cell stage. This "hamster test" has given rise to stories of Frankenstein dimensions of sinister laboratory experimentation on inter-species fertilization. It should be clearly understood that no attempt whatever is being made at cross-breeding. The only alternative would be to use human ova in the test, which in the first place can be obtained only by subjecting a woman to surgical invasion and in the second place would provoke the accusation of human embryo experimentation.

Many of us would agree with the magisterium of the Catholic church that infertility, however painful, must, like ill health, sometimes be accepted. Medical science does not have the answer to everything. It must be admitted too that the treatment of male infertility is usually disappointing, and the success rate with AIH is low.

What is not in doubt is that a couple who are desperate to have a child are very much better off if they can be told that there is no chance or virtually no chance of pregnancy, than to live from month to month in an agony of alternating hope and disappointment. They can then begin to make an adjustment to their lives or make plans for adoption.

Babies for adoption are scarce in Britain and the cut-off point with many adoption agencies is usually about 35 years for either of the prospective parents. There is nothing sadder than to see a couple go on hoping for a pregnancy until they find that they are too old for an adoption agency to consider them. For this reason alone it is worth making the diagnosis of male infertility.

In Vitro Fertilization

The achievement of IVF has so caught the public interest and imagination that it is being assumed here that most readers will have some acquaintance with the basic principles.

In about one-third of the cases of infertility in women the cause is blockage of the uterine tubes. This is often the result of previous pelvic inflammation, or endometriosis. Occasionally infertility in women is congenital, or an ectopic pregnancy may have necessitated surgical removal of the tube. It is sometimes suggested by opponents of IVF that women have blocked tubes more often than not as the result of previous abortion, sexually transmitted disease, or the use of the IUD, and that if the teaching of the Catholic church had been adhered to in the first place, the necessity for such difficult and morally dubious maneuvers would not have arisen.

This judgment is both erroneous and unfair. While all three practices may be capable of causing tubal infection, it can occur just as often after a spontaneous abortion that had to be completed by dilation and curettage; it is probably more common in fact because the whole process takes longer. Infection can follow a normal pregnancy and delivery; "one-child sterility" is widely recognized. It can result from appendicitis or any other cause of peritonitis. Also, tubal infection can occur *de nouveau* in a young woman who has never had sexual relations.

The first of my own patients to be assessed for possible IVF had widespread adhesions from pelvic appendicitis in her teens. At laparoscopy the ovaries were obscured by such dense and impenetrable adhesions that the case presented insuperable technical difficulties and she was rejected. At least she found out quite early in her marriage that conception was impossible and went on to adopt two children.

If the ovaries and uterus are healthy and functioning normally, the problem is the theoretically straightforward one of uniting sperm with ovum.

The "simple case" as originally conceived, involved obtaining, through a laparoscope, a ripe ovum from the surface of the woman's ovary at the time of natural ovulation. It was placed in a dish of nutrient medium together with the husband's sperm. If conditions were favorable, fertilization occurred and when the zygote reached the 4-to-8-cell stage it was placed in the uterine cavity where it was hoped it would successfully implant. In 1978, after years of work on the technique, the world's first "test-tube baby" was born in Britain and the achievement was almost universally acclaimed. It did not seem to offend any particular moral principle and it is widely believed that Pope John Paul I, while Patriarch of Venice, expressed his delight for the couple.

The procedure is theoretically simple, but the low success rate led to administering an ovulatory drug to the woman in the cycle preceding laparoscopy. By this means a number of ova can be produced and collected at one time and by exposing all of them to fertilization the chances of obtaining zygotes for implantation are greatly increased. Of those that appear microscopically to be dividing normally, 3 or 4 are arbitrarily selected and placed in the uterus with the hope that one of them will implant. As a result, the success rate is increasing to somewhere between 10 and 25 percent, depending largely on the experience and expertise of the operating team. In some centers unused embryos are frozen and stored for use in a further attempt if the first is unsuccessful, which is common. This saves precious hospital time and relieves the woman of the need for further surgery.

The fate of those spare embryos has since become central to the conflict about the morality of the whole procedure and was, in the UK, one of the main subjects for consideration by the Warnock Committee. This committee recommended that work on the human embryo should be permitted only under license and only up to the 14th day of development. The recommendations were largely adopted by the British Parliament in *The Human Fertilisation and Embryology Act of 1990.*

It would be of interest here to recall the comments of the various churches.

In the UK, the Roman Catholic Social Welfare Commission and Committee on Bio-Ethical Issues in their submissions to Warnock, tended to accept, though by no means unanimously, any IVF procedures that "had the settled intent of transferring each and every embryo to the maternal womb."[3] This would have serious medical drawbacks, however. IVF is time-consuming for both medical staff and patient, emotionally fraught for the couple, expensive, and much in demand. From the medical point of view, it would seem unfair to the patient and to others waiting for treatment to use anything other than a technique that has the highest chance of success. If ovulatory drugs are not used and only a single ovum is obtained, the expectation of success is greatly reduced. A further attempt would double the time, risk, and cost. On the other hand, if ovulatory drugs are used and many ova, perhaps 6-10 or more are obtained and successfully fertilized it is out of the question, for medical reasons, to implant them all, because multiple pregnancies carry a poor prognosis. The birth of sextuplets may make a good story in the media for a few days, but it is usually a tragedy for the parents. In 1987, sextuplets born prematurely after IVF to a childless couple in England died one by one over the space of 10 days and were a harrowing item on the nightly television news. Multiple implantation of up to 10 embryos has been carried out followed by selective reduction (destruction) at about the 8th week of pregnancy to reduce them to a manageable number. In the UK this has been condemned as unethical by the Royal College of Obstetricians and Gynecologists, which considers it one thing to leave a fertilized ovum in a dish and another to destroy it once it is implanted and developing normally. As one member of the College Ethics Advisory committee put it to me in a personal communication, "How would you like to feel that you had survived at the expense of your brothers and sisters?"

In the (Episcopal) Church of England in 1985, the Board of Social Responsibility accepted IVF with the rider that research using spare embryos up to 14 days—as recommended by Warnock—must be directed toward "worthy causes."[4]

The Board of the Church of Scotland in the same year was unhappy about any kind of embryo experimentation, although it was "not opposed to IVF as such."[5] This recommendation carries the inherent flaw that successful IVF—even in the "simple case"—depends on the years of experimentation that have made it possible. It opens wide the question of whether it is ever morally permissible to use information obtained by means which are themselves regarded as immoral.

In 1987 the Catholic church's Congregation for the Doctrine of the Faith issued its *Instruction in Respect of Human Life in Its Origins and on the Dignity of Procreation,* which to the dismay of some Catholics included condemnation of IVF in all circumstances, even the "simple case" that most people had expected to be approved.[6] It recalled the church's traditional opposition to masturbation even as a means of obtaining sperm, but its main objection to IVF was that it separated fertilization from the specific marital act. It maintained that an ovum had the right to be fertilized within the human body and that any other locus of fertilization offended the dignity of the human creative process.

In its submissions to Warnock on IVF the Catholic Committee on Bio-ethical Issues stated that it would not prohibit "procedures in which sperm and ovum are introduced, with or without prior mixing, into the womb."[7] It appears that a similar procedure might still be allowed with strict modifications, namely, that sperm and ovum are introduced separately without prior mixing, lest fertilization occur outside the body: GIFT—"gamete intrafallopian transfer." Also the sperm had to be obtained not by masturbation but from a condom that had been pierced with a hole beforehand.

After normal intercourse the sperm is viable for at least 48 hours, and fertilization can occur up to the end of this period. Chronologically, therefore, it need not be related to a specific marital act. It can take place either in the uterine tube or in the cavity of the uterus, which are hollow organs. The space within them is outside the body in the sense that it is separated from the mesomorphic cells which constitute the body proper by a layer of endothelium. Their cavity is continuous with the outside, like all other hollow organs.[8] The anatomical difference between fertilization in the uterine tube and fertilization in a dish is that of a few centimetres, and chronologically that of a few hours at most. These arguments smack of casuistry, and suggest that the magisterium appears to be ascribing a great deal of moral importance to an argument that will scarcely bear its weight. The object of the exercise is, after all, to enable a childless couple to fulfil their intense desire to produce a child of their own within the bond of matrimony.

Embryo Experimentation

The question of embryo experimentation has arisen as a side issue of IVF and, together with abortion, has generated more heat than any other bio-ethical issue in the last ten years. Occasionally this heat can be due to some misunderstanding of what is involved. It is in fact difficult to keep an embryo growing in a culture medium and it would die within a few weeks at most. It is, moreover, unlikely that even the most dedicated research worker would wish to proceed further. Only in horror fiction are babies actually grown in laboratories. By and large the medical profession does possess some sense of decency. The Warnock recommendation of a limit of 14 days seems to be acceptable to most research workers, and though it appears to have been somewhat arbitrarily selected it does coincide with the point at which the cleaving ovum begins visibly to differentiate into those cells that form the embryo proper and those that will form the placenta and amniotic sac. The word "pre-embryo" for an undifferentiated zygote is being widely and, to my mind, legitimately used. At 14 days it is only just visible to the naked eye.

For those who would accord full human right from fertilization onward, this recommendation and nomenclature will be totally unacceptable. They would point out that the embryo is no less alive and potentially human at 13 days than it is at 15 which is, of course, true. Three members of the Warnock Committee presented a minority report that opposed all embryo experimentation on the ground that while there could be no firm decision about when an embryo becomes a person, it has, from conception, a special status because of its potential for development to a stage at which everyone would accord it the status of a human person. This argument has been discussed in the chapter on the status of the embryo. Those who share this view would regard the *in vitro* destruction of an embryo, by allowing it to die or by destroying it at 14 days, to be in the same moral category as abortion. The term *"in vitro abortion"* is, in fact, used by some pro-life protagonists. The embryo is aborted in the strict biological sense of having been prevented from developing further, but neither the law pertaining to abortion nor the general understanding of it could be applied. In Britain the Infant Life (Preservation) Act refers to procuring a *miscarriage* and the Abortion Law Reform Act to terminating a *pregnancy*.[9] In the laboratory, because implantation has not taken place, there has been neither carriage nor pregnancy. Almost all research workers would agree, however, that the embryo must be regarded with respect as the ground material or blueprint of a human being, even if they would not go so far as to accord to it full human status and rights.

This view includes that of the Ethics Advisory Committee of the Royal College of Obstetricians and Gynaecologists of Britian and of the Church of England as expressed in its response to the Warnock Report.[10] Some members of the Church of England General Synod of 1985 pointed to a moral difference between using spare embryos adventitiously available as a by-product of IVF, and the direct production of embryos for the purpose of research.[11] Most of those who would allow research within limits agree that the cause must be worthy of the material being used and strictly monitored. This consideration also occupied a good deal of time in the Warnock inquiry.

In 1964, the Declaration of Helsinki laid down principles upon which all human experimentation should be conducted and pointed out a fundamental distinction between research conducted for the benefit of the person concerned, and research without direct diagnostic or therapeutic value to the person subjected to the research. It is the duty of the doctor, it added, to remain the protector of the life and health of that person, and it is essential to obtain valid consent for the experiment.

While the principles enshrined in this document are beyond reproach, they lead to immediate difficulties in the field of embryo research. The declaration refers to "person," but the personhood of the embryo is by no means universally recognized. Valid consent is meaningless in the same context and the only interpretation of it could be the consent of the parents as in the case of a minor. It is in fact mandatory to ask for donor consent from an IVF patient with regard to possible spare embryos. A woman undergoing a simple gynecological procedure such as diagnostic laparoscopy might give permission for an ovum to be removed at the same time for research purposes.

To limit embryological research to the strict aim of benefitting the embryo concerned would bring the whole program to a halt. Successful implantation of the first human embryo conceived *in vitro* followed years of research involving inevitable embryo loss before a successful technique was achieved.

Repeated failure to secure implantation is one of the most common causes of infertility, and a great deal of information on this subject has already been gained as a spin-off from IVF research. No doubt work will progress in this field as well as in genetics and in male subfertility. The ends can hardly be seen as anything but good, and for those who are sincerely doubtful about the means, a very delicate balance of conflicting priorities is set up. A theologian temperamentally opposed to compromising established teaching might see the problem in a very different light from a childless married woman who has suffered the heartbreak of repeated miscarriage. Her embryos have already all been lost and she would welcome any research that would give the next one a better chance.

There is a danger that if approval were to be given only to research that would benefit a particular embryo—if such a thing were possible—it would be logical to question the morality of a whole spectrum of medical work involving such well-established procedures as therapeutic trials.

For several years I worked in a surgical research unit attached to a university medical school. The project was related specifically to the problem of the resuscitation of severely shocked children. "Shocked" in this context means loss of circulating blood volume by hemorrhage, intestinal trauma, or extensive burns. As a team, we were engaged in serially measuring the blood volume of such children in order to establish a logical fluid replacement program. As a result of the work done, many children survived who would otherwise have died. Inevitably there were occasions when, in spite of our efforts, a child reached the stage of irreversible deterioration. We continued in such a case to monitor parameters such as blood volume, hemoconcentration, and renal function until the moment of death. Although it was emotionally harrowing, we did not consider such monitoring to be immoral. The amount of physical disturbance was kept to a minimum, but it could be argued that even that was impermissible. Sometimes a badly burned child was revived from the initial trauma only to die miserably several weeks later from skin loss and sepsis. This too could produce quite serious and painful self-doubt in those of us who were involved. Since then, new techniques in skin grafting and better control of infection have enabled such children to survive and return to normal living, but at the time we had to live with uncertainty and sometimes guilt. Those children would of course have died anyway. They were in our care because catastrophe had struck, which brings us to the proviso made by some contributors to the Church of England submissions to Warnock.

Those who consider limited embryo experimentation justified for the sake of the general good may restrict their acceptance to embryos adventitiously available as a by-product of IVF. Since they have not been produced for the purpose of experimentation, it can be viewed as an instance of the principle of double effect. The Warnock Committee took note of dissent on this point and recorded it in its report.

There is of course, no material difference between an embryo produced *in vitro* for the purpose of study and experimentation, and one adventitiously available. Their appearance and behavior are identical; an outside observer looking in a microscope would not be able to tell one from the other. Each has the same potential to become a human being and both require implantation to fulfill that potential.

I can see no middle way of regarding the question. If the potential to become a human person *ipso facto* bars the use of pre-embryos, then to make a distinction about how they came to be is irrelevant. If, on the other hand, the pre-embryo is regarded basically as a cluster of cleaving cells, human, but as yet human tissue rather than human being, their use for study and research for the advancement of medical science becomes permissible.

All cells from the same human body contain nuclei with an identical genetic pattern; this is what makes genetic fingerprinting possible in forensic investigation. Apart from the central nervous system, tissue cultures can be made from most body cells, although some are easier to grow than others. Embryonic cells are particularly valuable for study because of their large nuclei and rapid division; chromosomal activity can be observed from hour to hour.

All medical research must, of course, be subject to basic ethical principles. Suffering may not be intentionally caused, but if the embryo is as yet insensate no direct suffering *can* be caused. The donor has given consent and stands to benefit indirectly.

If these conditions have been satisfied, it would seem that the moral question hinges less on whether the embryo had been adventitiously or purposefully available than on the use to which it is put.

In all decision making, the intention and orientation of the decision maker is of paramount importance. For the believer it encompasses a sense of awareness of what comes from God. In genuine perplexity when the truth seems unknowable, the words of Brother Lawrence in *The Practice of the Presence of God* come to mind: "One must be careful to differentiate between the actions of the understanding and those of the will: the former are of little value and the latter all."[12]

Artificial Insemination by a Donor

DI attracts many legal and ethical complexities, but unlike IVF it is a simple technique with a high rate of success. For this reason it has been available at infertility clinics in Europe and North America for at least 40 years. The usual candidate is the fertile wife of an infertile husband, but it may be considered for use when the man is known to carry a dominant deleterious gene. The shortage of babies for adoption is almost certainly a factor in increasing the practice. Legally it is not regarded as adultery since there has been no sexual contact between the donor and the woman.

For the couple attending an infertility clinic it has the enormous social advantage of being an easily kept secret. Not even the closest of their family and friends need know that their successful pregnancy has come about through a third-party donor.

The Warnock recommendation was that at least basic information of ethnic origin and genetic health should be made available to the child at age 18, but it is not self-evident to my mind that it is in the child's best interests to be told of its origins. Adopting parents are invariably advised to tell their child the truth from the beginning and it presents few difficulties. To have been "chosen" by both mother and father is an easy and acceptable idea even to small children, but many parents would blanch at the thought of explaining DI to a three year old, even if it were thought to be desirable. If the truth is concealed until the child is old enough and sophisticated enough to understand it, which would probably be the early teens, it could well cause serious psychological trauma at an age when life within the family is often traumatic in any case. In British law at the moment there need not be anything on the birth certificate to reveal the child's origins; usually the social father registers the child as his own. To make this more acceptable psychologically and even legally, his semen is in some clinics mixed with that of the donor so that he could cling to the slight possibility that the child was indeed genetically his. On the whole, the Warnock recommendations seemed rather more concerned with the needs of the infertile couple than with those of the child. Most would agree, however, that as the practice of DI becomes more widespread, a tightening up of the law will be needed. Concerning the number of semen donations, for example, it has been estimated that in a population the size of that of Scotland (five million), 25 such donations could significantly raise the possibility of the chance of later incestuous matings.[13]

The guidelines for members of the Royal College of Obstetricians and Gynaecologists of Britain recommend that DI be performed only on a married woman and with the written consent of her husband. Since the doctor's role is by no means morally neutral, the guidelines are necessary. A minimal ethical demand would be that the doctor should have professional responsibility for ensuring that a child in whose conception he or she is involved will be born into a stable family environment. The right to have a child can never be absolute in that it involves interests other than those of the mother, although members of pressure groups for the rights of single women and lesbian couples would not perhaps agree.

The donors are most commonly medical students who are paid a small fee for their services. Warnock recommended that there should be a right to their anonymity, although it is obvious that some record must be kept and that it should be clearly understood that the donors would have neither parental rights nor responsibilities. They are screened for genetic defects and a record is kept of race and physical attributes such as stature and coloring.

In the Catholic submissions on DI to Warnock, the Social Welfare Commission advised that particular caution must be applied "where the risks involved something as fundamental to human life as the physical and social arrangements of fertility and as fundamental to the structure of society as the family."[14]

The Anglican (Episcopal) church response was, after debate, that a majority of their Social Responsibility Board agreed that DI was an acceptable practice for the married. The Board of the Presbyterian church of Scotland, on the other hand, was not prepared to support "the unwanted intrusion of a third party into the marriage."[15] This view was based to some extent on a previously published comment relating to the donor that the "deliberate separation of the responsibilities involved in sex, procreation, and parenting disrupted a set of relationships, physical, psychological, and spiritual, which together provide a rich soil for human identity and fulfillment."[16]

The Catholic comment seems curiously low-key compared with the severity of the strictures directed against IVF, strictures that would *de facto* prohibit it. Since 1987, of course, the statement of the Congregation for the Doctrine of the Faith has condemned on doctrinal grounds not only DI but all the other new fertility techniques.

While my sympathy for a childless couple is immense, I am not convinced that donor insemination is a desirable solution. The child of adoptive parents is genetically related to neither and has the same relationship to each; the parents can consider themselves equally responsible for the child and the way he or she turns out. The child born of IVF is the child of both parents in every sense. Children of both these groups are by definition "wanted"; their parents have gone to an unusual amount of trouble to have them, including submitting to professional scrutiny of their marriage. The parents in the case of DI have also very much wanted a child, but this child is an offspring of the mother, not of the "father." He, in fact, is a stepfather, which is an inherently tricky relationship.

There must be few natural parents who have not asked themselves at times where one or other of their children got a particularly disagreeable characteristic. This question must be acute and potentially painful in the case of DI. There are difficult times in any family and there must be inevitable conjecture about what manner of man the father was. Even if the child graduates *summa cum laude,* the natural family pride of the father may be a little dampened by the thought that the child's inherent brilliance has nothing to do with him. If all these difficulties are surmountable, there remains the difficult decision of whether, what, how, and when to tell the child of its true parentage.

We may wonder what kind of person becomes a donor. The fee is purposely very small so that the incentive cannot be financial; most donors probably regard it as analogous to the giving of a pint of blood in that the donor has no personal contact or knowledge of the recipient. However, the donation and acceptance of anonymous sperm to produce a child has a highly charged emotional content which is absent from giving or receiving a blood transfusion.

The stance of the Catholic church on contraception has been

questioned elsewhere in this book. A loving and continuing sexual relationship without the necessity of procreation is in my opinion easily acceptable in a way that procreation without the necessity for a relationship is not, more with regard to the donor than to the recipient.

In John Steinbeck's play *Burning Bright*, the woman contrives a brief, and for her, distasteful sexual relationship with a younger man in order to give a child to the husband she loves. In the end she is ready to kill her lover for threatening to tell him. Doing what she did is not recommended as a solution for the wives of infertile men, but it may in some ways be more human than DI.

By now, there must be many children born of DI, but by the very delicacy that forbids their identification a follow-up study of their subsequent family history is precluded. Without the possibility of reassurance of this nature I am reluctant to recommend DI to a childless couple, however deeply I sympathize with their great desire for a child.

Surrogate Motherhood

Surrogate motherhood is not new, as we can see by examining the lineage of many noble families, or even Scripture (Genesis 16:1-3). "Sarai, Abram's wife, bore him no children. She had an Egyptian maid whose name was Hagar, and Sarai said to Abraham: 'Behold, now the Lord has prevented me from having children. Go in to my maid Hagar, it may be that *I* shall have children by her.'" Sarai's use of the first person starkly reflects the outlook of patrilinear societies on the role of women in furthering the race.

Surrogate motherhood is the reverse of DI in that genetically the child is that of the father but not of the social mother. It has attracted much more public attention and reprobation because it is not only done but by its nature can be observed. Even with the comparatively modern refinement of artificial insemination a woman cannot easily conceal a pregnancy. Ovum donation would be a more exact biological equivalent to SM, but apart from any ethical considerations, which would be comparable to those of

DI, this latter is technically challenging and the indications are few.

Among the causes of female infertility ovarian failure *per se* is comparatively rare. Much more often, apart from the common one of tubal blockage, the cause of infertility in women is associated with implantation problems and with the inability to carry the pregnancy to term. If a woman's own fertilized ova repeatedly fail to implant, it is unlikely that a donated one will do so. If the problem is poor maternal health, the pregnancy would be equally difficult.

Two interesting cases were reported in 1987. In one, a woman with a healthy uterus whose ovaries had been removed because of cystic disease successfully carried to term a pregnancy resulting from IVF, in which the ovum had been donated by her sister. In the case of sisters the genetic pool is similar, and, since the host mother was able to carry the child, a normal bonding relationship was established. The donor sister had, of course, to submit to treatment with ovulatory drugs and to ovum collection, but in the close and loving family relationship that seemed to exist this did not present a problem. The circumstances were unusual, and unlikely to be repeated except on a very small scale. The exact obverse would be sperm donation by the brother of an infertile man. It would be simple and more than likely it has been done, but it would not be material for medical or popular reporting.

The other case involved the twin sister of an infertile woman. The fertility problem was the more common one of healthy ovaries but with the inability to conceive and carry a pregnancy. The ovum of the childless woman was fertilized *in vitro* by her husband's sperm, then implanted in the uterus of her sister who carried it to term, gave birth, and returned the baby to its genetic parents. The generosity required of the sister was of a very high order. Not only did she accept the discomfort and hazards of pregnancy and delivery, but she faced the emotional hurdle of detaching herself from the newborn child to give it back to its genetic mother.

A foreign embryo might be thought likely to provoke a rejection response in the manner of a donated kidney, but could be expected to be less of a problem between sisters. Furthermore, a baby conceived naturally need not inherit its mother's blood group and tissue type, so it may be that there is in nature some natural suppression of this immune response during pregnancy. Whatever the technical, moral, and legal problems, it seems unlikely that this technique would be considered for more than a very small number of infertile women.

Although the Warnock Committee recognized the genetic distinction between "womb leasing" as just described, and surrogate motherhood as it is commonly understood, it was generally biased toward a social rather than biological view of parenthood. This is similar to its evaluation of donor insemination. Its recommendation was, in general, that the act of carrying a fetus from implantation to full term should be regarded as conferring true motherhood on a woman, and that it was difficult to see any legal circumstances in which this right would be challenged.

The right has, of course, been challenged since Warnock. In a long and widely reported legal battle in the United States the commissioning couple were eventually awarded the right of claim to a baby born of a surrogate mother who had changed her mind about handing over the baby.

The possibility of such conflicting claims with their distasteful publicity and heartbreak for parents and child led the Warnock committee to recommend that to use the services of a carrying mother should be a criminal offense. This was to apply to private agencies arranging such matters, whether profit-making or non-profit, and the recommendations were later adopted in the British Embryo Bill. The bill was in accord with a statement in the *Journal of Medical Ethics* in 1981 by W.J. Winslade: "The principle has a potential for economic exploitation, moral confusion, psychological harm in the surrogate mothers, the prospective adoptive parents, and the children."[17]

When all the moral, social, and legal difficulties of both DI and

SM are considered, it would seem to many people that money and resources might well be put to less dubious use, such as funding an organization that would tackle, for example, the legal difficulties of adopting an orphan from another country. Enthusiasm for research in new reproductive technology has almost certainly been fueled in Europe by the shortage of babies for adoption.

It could be said that there is no such thing as an unwanted child. A woman with an unwanted pregnancy would find no shortage of adoptive parents, but many childless couples who would eagerly adopt find themselves at the bottom of a waiting list so long that they fear they will be too old to be eligible by the time they reach the top. It may seem to be ironic too that in many countries other children may die while waiting for life-saving treatment in hospitals hampered by understaffing or lack of money, or that research into common causes of childlessness such as recurrent abortion may be limited by dependence on uncertain charitable funding.

Chapter 9

Homosexuality and Aids

I believe none of the mainstream Christian churches would find themselves in disagreement with Cardinal Hume of Westminster who, in an interview in 1987, linked the disaster of Chernobyl with the AIDS crisis. The first disaster forces us to consider what we are doing with our human environment; the second, our attitude to human relations and sexual behavior in particular. Nor would these churches disagree that advocating the use of condoms could be seen as a counsel of despair. None of the churches condones sexual promiscuity, whether heterosexual or homosexual, and all would urge self-control, fidelity, and restraint as being most in accord with human dignity and Christian ideals. The Catholic church, while fully sharing these views, also has a high tradition of realistic recognition of human frailty and a particular emphasis on the doctrine of forgiveness, which underlies its very possession of a special sacrament of reconciliation. The gospel we read with such reverence and emphasis proclaims this truth; no one is beyond the pale.

It is clear that the angst of the widely reported conference of Catholic bishops in 1986 on the use of the condom as an AIDS protective was based primarily on the thorny question of contraception. Were the protective to be a vaccine or an antibiotic, it seems that their concern would be less, or at least different. The fact that a condom is also a contraceptive seems to be the central cause of concern, since they suggested that its use might just possibly be morally acceptable in a case where conception is impossible, for example, when the wife is pregnant or past childbearing.

In the homosexual relationship, contraception is not an issue, but the bishops—wisely, I think—did not address this question, though it is plainly an urgent one: is a homosexual relationship made *more* sinful if protection is taken against transmitting a deadly disease?

Consider the normal heterosexual situation and try to apply the bishops' thinking within the framework of normal living. It was their view that if a man has been exposed in any manner to the risk of AIDS, he may not use a condom to protect his legal wife unless conception is for some reason impossible. But what if she is using the "safe period," which is not really safe, or lactation, which is only partly safe, or on the pill or sterilized, which are wholly safe, like pregnancy, but are themselves unlawful in the eyes of the church? The permutations and grades of moral uncertainty are mind-boggling and at the end of the day the ordinary Catholic may wonder what it is all about.

It must be remembered with regard to these strictures that AIDS can be acquired unwittingly by blood transfusion, by treatment for hemophilia, or by an infected needle, especially in countries where the disease is endemic. Travelers to such countries are now advised to take a small supply of hypodermic needles in case of illness while abroad. The HIV can be detected in the blood long before symptoms of the disease appear, if they ever do, and it seems unreasonable to forbid people to take steps to protect at least their marriage partner.

Homosexuality is a difficult problem for any doctor, and especially for the Catholic doctor, when the teaching of the magisterium is so specifically—and so distressingly—reiterated.

In fairness to the church it must be said that while it may condemn all homosexual practice, there is within it a body of pastoral concern for the individual. It is my experience, like that of many other doctors and clergy, that when faced with a person with a homosexual problem, rather than with the problem of homosexuality, or in considering a couple in an established homosexual relationship, the situation is viewed in an entirely different light.

Compassion and sympathy must be especially felt for a Catholic who may already be heavily guilt-ridden, yet feels trapped by his or her sexual bias.

All mammalian species have non-reproductive members; in the human they are estimated to number about ten percent of the population. It is almost certain that homosexual tendencies like so many other tendencies have a genetic basis that may be reinforced by psychological factors in the familial and social environment. Its common association with artistic ability has often been noted; people who are gifted in the arts tend in the nature of things to associate with one another professionally and socially in a circle which by its very nature tends to be accepting and tolerant. The fact that homosexual relationships arise in this and similar environments should cause little surprise. Few people, though, would condone homosexual promiscuity any more than they would condone heterosexual promiscuity.

As a counselor with a national organization, I have been involved from time to time with clients with homosexual problems that were sufficiently severe to bring them to the point of despair, often from excessive guilt rather than open homosexual practice, as the following cases illustrate.

A man of about 35, successful in business, with a wife and three children had become obsessed by his inability to pass urine in a public washroom. He felt the problem was so ludicrous that he had great difficulty in referring to it and had never been able to tell it to anyone, including his wife and family doctor. It had reached the point when he was leaving his office at half-hour intervals to go to the public washroom merely to see if he could "manage," and this was causing considerable curiosity and consternation among his co-workers. He had stopped going out socially in the evening in case his male friends should detect and remark on his difficulty, and had been unable to explain this to his wife, even though his unsociability was causing friction between them.

In other respects he maintained he was happily married. He had been the younger of two boys and his elder brother, whom he described as "big and macho," had constantly made disparaging remarks in their youth about his younger brother's smaller genitalia, suggesting that he was "girlish and queer." He had never had a physical homosexual relationship but was convinced that his brother's insinuations were justified and that his apparently successful marriage was a sham.

He gradually came to terms with the reality of the situation and made a remarkable improvement.

In the following instance a man, who was older, did less well.

A married man in his early fifties with a grown-up family of two had gone through a difficult period when the children left home and he and his wife were thrown back on one another's company. They had married fairly late and had previously considered themselves to be suitably and happily matched. The recent friction had made him severely depressed and had re-opened intense guilt feelings from his youth that he had thought were buried. He had been brought up as a Catholic, and as a boy of about 14 had confessed to his parish priest a strong physical attraction to an older boy at school. This had been very badly handled by his confessor, who without further inquiry or follow-up had impressed upon him the seriousness and dire consequences of such a mortal sin. The physical contact had been minimal, but from that moment he had secretly labeled himself homosexual. When his marriage was in transient difficulty 40 years later, he took the whole burden of guilt upon himself: "I should not have married; I should never have had children." Although he improved and the marriage in time settled down, I do not think he was ever fully persuaded of his innocence.

Homosexuality is one of the most common sexual variants. Some workers in the field would distinguish between homosexuality, which would be applied only to cases of established and long-standing physical sexual activity, and homophilia for cases where the tendencies are confined to friendships of only a mildly erotic nature.[1] Also, heterosexual men can display temporary homosexual behavior in certain restrictive conditions: old-fashioned boys' boarding schools, prolonged service in the military, and prisons being the most obvious examples.

In Britain, before the change in the law following the Wolfenden Report (Sexual Offenses Act, 1967) which permitted male homosexual practices by two consenting adults in private, openly homosexual men were subject to ostracism, gossip, and sometimes blackmail by the rest of society. A writer of the caliber of E. M. Forster, a homosexual, felt unable to publish much of his work in his lifetime. Secondary psychological problems often followed, and suicide was not uncommon among homosexuals.

Homosexual women are less inclined to be promiscuous and often settle down to a happy, more or less permanent relationship. The AIDS problem does not of course arise. There is no legal regulation on the matter of artificial insemination by a donor, but the Royal College of Obstetricians and Gynaecologists recommends to its members that it should not be considered, a view generally shared by the Warnock Committee.

Society at the moment seems to be going through a period of exaggerated revolt against the stern and judgmental view of homosexuality that was the norm a generation ago. It would not be an overstatement to say that the life of the man in the second case just quoted had been ruined by guilt over something that had been no more than a schoolboy crush on an older boy, a guilt so entrenched that subsequent (though delayed) marriage and fatherhood had been unable to eradicate it.

Such crushes in both girls and boys in their teens are so common that they can be regarded as part of normal sexual development. Provided excessive guilt is not implanted, most teenagers soon grow out of them, especially if they are allowed a prudent and healthy amount of contact with the opposite sex.

Sadly, overreaction to the harsh views of thirty years ago almost certainly underlies the current elevation of male homosexuality to a fashionable cult. The association with drugs, especially—on the American continent—cocaine, and the use of highly advertised and glamorized "aphrodisiacs" has given rise to a culture of homosexual excess which is debasing and highly disturbing. The epidemic of AIDS in such an environment and now spreading far beyond it will force us, as Cardinal Hume rightly stated, to take stock of our human relations and the whole area of sexual education and behavior.

The epidemic of AIDS may in time cause a reversion to the pre-Wolfenden attitude of the public to homosexual men: with increasing interest in child sexual abuse, for instance, homosexual men are commonly viewed as posing a greater risk to children, but as more and more evidence is documented, this erroneous belief is more obviously exposed.[2]

Now that HIV infection is becoming more widespread throughout society and can be contracted by heterosexual contact as well as by accidental, non-sexually related causes, there is an increasing measure of sympathy for the victims. Hospices for the care of AIDS patients are widely supported.

The fact, however, that the disease appeared originally (in the West) among homosexual men has given it a stigma greater than that associated with other sexually transmitted diseases; also it is incurable at present. Suggestions for a screening program, therefore, provoke an emotional response and understandable alarm.

A different view might be taken by those involved in medical practice and epidemiology. For as long as I can remember, pregnant women have had their blood screened routinely for syphilis and gonorrhea at their first prenatal visit, along with blood group, rh-factor, and the like. These comprise a routine battery of tests fed into a computer. It never occurred to me specifically to tell a prenatal patient that her blood would be tested for syphilis.

A case can certainly be made for adding HIV testing to the list of routine screening procedures in ante-natal clinics, hospital admission departments, or in any other circumstances in which routine blood tests are customarily made. Apart from its diagnostic value, it seems reasonable to protect obstetric staff and surgical teams. A surgeon uses sharp instruments when operating and there is a fair amount of blood around at the most normal birth. Infected blood could put at risk not only the nursing and medical attendants at the delivery, but the porters and domestic staff who handle and dispose of the placenta, pathological material, and soiled linen. The baby of an infected mother could also be at risk and in need of special care. If the test is done, I can see no alternative to informing the patient of a positive result.

To return to the attitude of church and society to homosexuality, the Church of England in synod conferences has at times aroused passionate dissent among its members by deliberating openly on the position of homosexual priests when the matter could perhaps more suitably have been left to the discretion of individual bishops. An occasional Episcopalian vicar will scandalize many people by conducting a "marriage" between homosexual men or women. On the other hand, there has been angry reaction on both sides of the Atlantic to the Vatican statement of July 1992, counseling against legislation for the protection of the civil rights of homosexuals. Many viewed the document as further evidence of the chronic inability of the Congregation for the Doctrine of the Faith to understand and come to terms with the realities of human sexuality.

It would be better if all the Christian churches could bring themselves to regard the existence of homosexuality and in particular of steady established homosexual relationships as a fact of life and a private matter, neither remarking nor condoning nor judging, but accepting in a spirit of Christian generosity.

Chapter 10

Death and Dying

For all the current search for an accurate and acceptable definition, the diagnosis of death in ordinary circumstances is not difficult.

A relative tending a dying patient at home will tell the doctor
the exact time to the minute that the patient died during the night.
On a cremation certificate this time has to be stated and most doctors do not hesitate to rely on such evidence, or on that of a nurse
if the patient dies in the hospital. It is customary for the doctor to
examine the body, and, in the case of cremation, obligatory, but
the placing of the stethoscope on the chest is more a ritual than a
necessity. It is common to be called to a car accident and be told
by the ambulance driver or police officer that one casualty is badly injured and that the other is dead. A confirmatory glance is
usually enough. Since so many of the populace die in the hospital,
or in nursing homes, however, many people may reach middle
age without having seen a dead person. The classical family
deathbed scene with its last words and solemn leave-taking is almost a thing of the past.

In the public mind advances in medicine have almost called
into question the inevitability of death; this is understandable
when, for example, a common, potentially fatal condition like
congestive cardiac failure can be brought so easily under control
and the patient restored to many more years of normal living. It is
not surprising that people think there is a cure for nearly everything. Often doctors and nurses themselves have unreal expecta-
tions and have a feeling of defeat and even guilt when medical
science fails. To follow the general principle of safeguarding life

is, of course, a good general basis for the conduct of medical practice, but every doctor will be called upon many times in professional life to judge when to "give in" and let nature take its course. This consists almost always of ceasing to strive to keep the patient alive, but the circumstances vary so widely that there can be no field of decision making more suited to the thoughtful application of situation ethics. A typical example in my experience in the case of the aged is the following:

> An old woman of 96 in a geriatric nursing home was frail and tired both in mind and body and had often expressed her longing for a peaceful death. She developed, quite suddenly, gangrene in the leg. She could have been transferred to a general hospital and had the leg amputated, an operation she would almost certainly have survived with modern anesthesia. The broncho-pneumonia that would have resulted from immobilization could have been treated with a battery of antibiotics. In the event, after consultation with the nursing staff and the relatives, it was decided to keep her where she was, among people she knew, and to control any pain with morphine. She died peacefully after a week.

In the younger patient with advanced malignant or other disease the decision can be more difficult, but the principles of treatment initiated by the hospice movement are being rapidly assimilated into the community, and, if the provision of specially trained nurses becomes adequate, dying at home may again become more common.

Sometimes the circumstances can be less straightforward as in the following case.

> A 50-year-old patient who was overweight and a heavy smoker was admitted to a general hospital for an exploratory laparotomy. During the operation an advanced bowel tumor was found which had already invaded the liv-

er, and the abdomen was closed without further surgery. After the operation she developed a chest infection, which is very common after upper abdominal surgery, especially in smokers and the obese. For this she was treated with strenuous physiotherapy to promote coughing and expectoration. She found this so distressing that when she was discharged after a few days to convalesce under my care she begged to be left alone. She was an intelligent woman who had guessed, from the evasive answers she had been given in the immediate post-operative period, that she had an inoperable condition. We had always had an excellent relationship and after a calm and honest discussion with her I decided to agree to her request. The family fully agreed and she died, predictably, about two weeks later of broncho-pneumonia, requiring very little in the way of sedation.

It has been truly said that it is one thing to prolong life and another to prolong dying.[1]

Sometimes, in an emergency, life-saving measures have to be instituted in circumstances where the consequences cannot be calculated. The two following examples will illustrate this.

A young man of 22 was severely injured when his car skidded into a ditch on an icy road. On examination at the scene of the accident he was found to be deeply unconscious, very blue, and breathing only intermittently. The heart, however, was still beating. He was intubated at the roadside and taken to a hospital in an ambulance that was equipped with a hand ventilator. He remained in a deep coma for three weeks and then made a complete recovery except for minor loss of visual field. If this man had sustained severe, permanent brain damage there might have been reason later to regret the resuscitative measures that had been taken in the emergency.

An urgent call was received to attend to a child of 8 who had been found unconscious in a stand of trees with a rope around his neck. He had been playing cowboys with some playmates and it was they who raised the alarm. A passing postman had released the rope and summoned help. On examination he looked dead, with blue lips and widely dilated pupils but the heart was still beating erratically. Mouth to mouth respiration was immediately started but in spite of this procedure, combined with external cardiac massage, the heartbeat faltered more and more and eventually stopped. After about 6 minutes both measures were discontinued, since it was considered that severe brain damage must by then be irreversible.

These two cases illustrate the physiological interdependence of the respiratory center in the brain-stem and the heart, which can continue beating independently after brain-stem injury, provided it has an adequate supply of oxygen from the lungs. The respiratory center itself depends on oxygenated blood being pumped by a functioning heart. In the first case above, the respiratory center in the brain was damaged in the injury and this initiated a downward spiral by interfering with the respiratory function on which it depended for its own oxygen supply. The heart has its own built-in pacemaker and in a young person it might continue to beat for 10 to 20 minutes in such circumstances until it too runs out of oxygen. Luckily for this young man, ventilation could be started before this happened and the brain injury proved later to be recoverable after surgical decompression.

In the case of the little boy, brain-stem injury had been severe from the time of injury (proven subsequently by post-mortem examination). Central nervous system cells are irreplaceable; the quota for each human person and each part of the brain is finite. The presence of a heartbeat justified attempts at resuscitation in the emergency, but spontaneous respiration never occurred and the heart eventually failed to respond to stimulation. It had been hopeless from the beginning, but impossible to make such a judgment immediately.

In the case of a heart attack, the chain of interdependence of heart-lungs-respiratory center is broken at a different link. The respiratory center is itself undamaged until it fails secondarily after a few minutes from lack of oxygen. If the heart can be restarted within this time by mechanical or electrical stimulation, breathing will usually recommence. If the heart is damaged by a massive infarction, it is unlikely to continue to beat spontaneously, but often, if the damage is less severe, death is caused by ventricular arrhythmia which is reversible. Speed is everything in such a case. Such emergencies occur frequently enough both in family and in hospital practice and every case has to be judged on its merits; many people recover from it. About 20 years ago in a large city hospital a general recommendation was made by the administrator that defibrillators were not to be used on patients over the age of 65. This caused such outrage among the medical staff and general public that it was hastily withdrawn—and rightly so.

Extraordinary Means

General rules in this area of patient care are totally inappropriate as the following case demonstrates.

A colleague in medical practice was training for a postgraduate qualification. This involved several years of rotation through different hospitals and hospital departments. While she was working in hematology she had a patient severely ill with terminal leukemia, a woman in her late thirties with a husband and two schoolage children. Both the patient and family accepted the inevitability of a fatal outcome, and a very good relationship was established between them and the medical staff. The doctor was in Intensive Care one day and was aghast to be presented with this patient, now unconscious, who had been transferred to the unit for intubation and ventilation. The doctor refused to do it, and had it not been for the backing of a senior colleague she might well have incurred disciplinary censure severe enough to end her medical career.

Similar incidents are widely reported elsewhere. It is true that the term "extraordinary means" of treatment so long used by the Christian churches no longer includes simple ventilation, but the phrase is in any case unsatisfactory since it tends to focus on the type of treatment given rather than on the patient. Intubation and ventilation were indicated and proved to be life saving in the case of the young man who was severely injured in the accident, but the same procedure would have been totally inappropriate in the case just above. They would have been "extraordinary" in the latter case, but not in the former. Rules are certainly not the answer, although it is true that to advocate judging every case on its merits is to place a heavy burden on the individual doctor. Mistakes are inevitably made and recognized only with hindsight. It takes a certain amount of moral courage to risk being wrong.

Congenital Abnormality

This is a particularly difficult area. Exact neo-natal assessment is not always easy and the mother is emotionally shocked and vulnerable. Sometimes babies born with Down's Syndrome have an associated cardiac anomaly which may be severe as we see in the following case:

A baby who was the fourth in an otherwise normal family was born with Down's Syndrome. She had a severe cardiac abnormality and required treatment for cardiac failure almost from birth. The heart lesion was not considered to be operable and in the three years of her life she became more and more frequently ill with associated lung infections. She required constant re-admissions to a pediatric hospital and this greatly distressed her. Finally, after consultation with the devoted parents, the pediatrician decided to treat the next episode of broncho-pneumonia with nursing care only, at home, and in the end she died after a very short illness.

The decision was taken not because she had Down's Syndrome, but because her cardiac failure had become intractable.

Babies suffering from uncomplicated Down's Syndrome should be regarded as having the same rights as other children: an intercurrent infection would be treated with the same vigor. In the UK, there was a widely reported case in 1981 involving the parents of a Down's baby who refused permission for an operation to relieve an intestinal obstruction in the child. The surgeon successfully applied to make the child a ward of the court and the necessary permission was obtained. The view of both the court and the surgeon was that the child's life after the operation would be in no way intolerable but simply be that of any other Down's infant.[2] Few doctors would disagree with this conclusion.

I have only limited experience of thalidomide babies. Many, with the aid of modern technology, devoted care, and determination have succeeded in living tolerable lives.

The following baby was severely affected.

A child was born without incident in our local maternity unit, the last of a family of five. The mother had a previous history of nervous breakdown, but had been well throughout this pregnancy. Later she remembered that early in pregnancy she had taken, for a few nights only, the remaining few tablets of a night sedative which had been prescribed for her by the psychiatric hospital several years earlier, when the dire effect of thalidomide on the embryo was yet unknown. Thalidomide had been thought indeed to be the perfect sedative with a very low toxicity. The baby was totally without arms or legs and also had an extremely small head with tiny eyes. It breathed on delivery but was never vigorous. The mother did not wish to see it and asked, quite reasonably under the circumstances, to be discharged the following day to look after her other children. The baby was lovingly nursed by the staff and offered drinks of warm sweetened water only, for comfort. These were mostly regurgitated and the baby died after two days. It seemed likely that it had narrowing of the esophagus as well as all the other abnormalities. Surgical correction of this latter condition is a major undertaking, even in an otherwise healthy baby, and referral to a surgical unit was not contemplated here.

The degree of disability in spina bifida babies varies enormously but without closure of the defect the child will die of infection. Most neuro-surgeons have a grading system for assessing operability. If the findings are truly marginal and the final decision is left to the parents they require a good deal of support, whichever way they decide. Those who decide to have nothing done are probably the more vulnerable and are greatly helped if the family doctor or surgeon strongly reassures them that they have made the right decision, whatever his own personal feelings might be. Guilt is very common after such an agonizing choice and is easier for the parents to bear if it is shared in this way.

The Aged Person

Guilt may also be a problem with the family of a seriously ill aged relative, perhaps with pneumonia following a stroke. The doctor might very obliquely seek the family feeling, but if it is clear that their inclination is to let the patient die in peace, it is my opinion that in such a case they should be left with the impression that they are agreeing with the doctor, rather than the other way around. A devoted daughter might say she would "never forgive herself" if she thought she was hastening her aged mother's death, and it seems unfair to lay this whole burden on someone who is already emotionally overwrought. I accept, however, that this personal viewpoint may well be considered to be against a general trend toward encouraging people to make their own decisions and take full responsibility for their actions in all areas of life.

Telling the Patient

There is a welcome general bias now toward telling the patient the truth, an attitude widely held in the United States. There is no doubt in my mind that this is a better way than evasion, and in ℮ case of malignant disease the sooner the patient is told the better. If patients have a lump that might be malignant and they are told right away, they and the doctor can tackle the problem together, stage by stage. Respect for personhood is basic here. The following case illustrates this point.

A man of 30, married with two children, came with a lump in the testicle and I suspected a malignant condition from the first examination. He had hoped for reassurance but the possibility of malignancy had been in his own mind. He was referred for biopsy which confirmed a testicular tumor and he was told of the report immediately. He was also told that while such tumors can be highly malignant, they are also very sensitive to radiation and chemo-therapy. He required a long course of both and had a very bad time, being miserably nauseated for days at home after each weekly outpatient treatment over about a year. He lost all his hair and became anemic, but bore it all with great fortitude. He was greatly helped by his wife who had been fully in the picture from the beginning and encouraged him when his spirits drooped from time to time. Because he had been told the truth from the very first, they knew the treatment was lifesaving and there is little doubt that this kept them going. He made a complete recovery and remains well many years later.

Except for a few patients known to be unable to cope with psychological pressure, this policy of telling the patient early is the one of choice. Too many patients used to come out of the hospital after an operation for an "ulcer," or something equally vague, and were totally unprepared for possible deterioration as in the following case.

A single, well-educated professional woman came with symptoms suggesting appendicitis. A mass, which was easily felt in the right lower abdomen, seemed almost certain to be an appendix abscess. I sent her to the hospital and the surgeon agreed with the diagnosis. He treated her conservatively with antibiotics as an in-patient for ten days, and planned to re-admit her three months later for appendectomy, by which time the inflammatory process would have settled. This is the usual procedure in such a case. Just before discharge she suddenly developed intestinal obstruction requiring urgent operation. Unfortunately, the mass was not an appendix abscess but a tumor of the bowel with secondary deposits in the liver. The obstruction was bypassed and she was, for some reason, not told the truth; most probably the emergency surgeon had not been the one in overall charge of the case. When she came home she was perplexed and frustrated by her slow convalescence and fretted about getting back to work, though she admitted she did not feel up to it. It fell to me to tell her the truth, which was, in fact, a great relief to her. She had always thought herself to be physically and mentally tough, as indeed she was, and the true diagnosis now explained her failure to recuperate. She faced further deterioration unflinchingly and a few months later died peacefully under my care in our local hospital.

If the truth is told early enough it can be coupled with hope and encouragement. With few exceptions not to tell patients the truth seems to be robbing them of their very dignity, and if it is not done at the beginining it is very difficult to do so later on.

Meantime a process of systematic deception is set up between doctor and patient, often involving the closest members of the family. It is very sad, in what has been a good marriage, when one spouse insists on deceiving the other to the very end. The patient, who will probably have his own suspicions, must feel very alone facing the most awesome part of his life; his wife, with whom he had previously discussed everything, is not available at the end. Sometimes a circle of deception is set up when he does not wish to distress her by telling her that he knows, and she assumes a false cheerfulness which is painful for them both. The doctor who participates in such a deception loses not only the trust of the patient but of the rest of the family when they have had time to think about it and when they themselves fall ill.

Even when the outlook is bleak the patient usually benefits from being told the truth. Most of us, probably, fear dying more than death and if the truth has been told, assurance can be given of good care and adequate pain relief when it is needed. While totally avoiding the direct imposition of his religious beliefs upon a patient, the doctor who has a religious basis in his own life and work might well ask as he walks up the garden path for his daily visit that God should, in the words of the hymn, be that day in his head and in his understanding, in his mouth and in his speaking. If it is appropriate, the priest or minister can be involved from the beginning rather than at the end as the herald of death, as has been so often the case in the past. In such circumstances, if it can be achieved, a good doctor-clergy relationship can be of immeasurable benefit to all concerned.

The Management of the Aged

Advances in medical care coupled with a generally rising standard of living have brought about a dramatic increase in the numbers of aged people in the populace. In the UK about one-fifth of all admissions to National Health Service hospitals is of people over the age of 75; such patients usually have multiple pathology and their hospital stay is therefore more likely to be prolonged.

Since the stock of brain cells in each person is finite, the number of old people suffering from some degree of confusion will rise concomitantly with increasing life-expectancy.

As every doctor knows, once an old person has been in a hospital for a prolonged period it is very difficult to resettle them in the community. It can be a major problem to find a suitable place for an old person who no longer needs hospital care but is not fit enough to live alone at home. Grown-up children have an obligation to care for elderly parents, but we should not presume that the parents will not resent this dependence on a son or daughter. One of the best investments health and social services could make would be to fund and encourage simple measures to help old people to stay in their own homes. Illich (1975) argues for a refocusing on the priorities of health care: "Dependence on professional intervention tends to impoverish the non-medical health-supporting and healing aspects of the social and physical environment."[3]

Local authorities who are forced to economize on their home services simply provoke an increased demand for nursing home accommodation or hospital care, which is very much more expensive. Apart from the economic factor, most old people prefer to live at home, and it would be reasonable to ask, when a move to a nursing home is being contemplated, whether it is for the real benefit of the elderly person concerned. It is questionable if even moderate dementia is sufficient ground to take them out of their home, as long as they are reasonably safe and reasonably nourished.

Many old people live in contented confusion and dubious hygiene, perhaps with a cat or dog. For many years I visited an old lady who, once her few medical problems had been disposed of, was always eager to chat over a cup of coffee. The mug was cursorily wiped with the floor cloth she used to clean up after the cat but neither of us ever came to any harm, and I always looked forward to her sharp and witty comments on current affairs. She invariably slept with her feet on the pillow and her head at the bottom of the bed for the very good reasons that the pillow elevated her swollen ankles and this arrangement also gave her a view of the birds she fed at the window. She was considered by some to be quite seriously demented.

Although a patient like this may worry family, friends, and neighbors, moving her to a "home," however cleaner, warmer, and safer, is not necessarily in the old person's best interests. Money is well spent on home services, meals on wheels, and centers where the old person who is just managing at home can go occasionally to have a bath and other necessary bodily attention. The right of such a person to stay at home can be strongly defended on human grounds, even if it is conceded that they are at some personal risk.

When a doctor should treat and not treat a demented old person can be a difficult problem since the line defining mental competence is likely to be indistinct. Intellectual impairment is uneven and an old person who is confused about day-to-day matters may have well-considered opinions about her future. It is a case for individual judgment and often the only thing to do is to try to discern from previous knowledge of the person what he or she would be likely to choose. This applies not only to treatment but to medical diagnosis.

If a frail old woman in her nineties becomes anemic, one would suspect that she might be bleeding from some part of her gastro-intestinal tract. A barium x-ray examination is not too uncomfortable, but endoscopy certainly is. If anything were to be found such as cancer of the colon, would she want or be able to tolerate an operation? Hospital diagnostic departments themselves are confusing and frightening to old people. If a tumor were to cause an acute obstruction, an operation would be indicated at once to relieve distress, but apart from the possibility of this emergency, might it not be better to let her fade away quietly and peacefully from anemia? The answer must be that sometimes it would and sometimes it wouldn't, and one can only hope for the grace to make the right decisions most of the time.

Respect for personhood is the overriding consideration in the treatment of the aged. It is doubtful, if ever ethical, to remove an old person from his home against his will for the sake of peace of mind of neighbors, social workers, or a concerned family. Their criteria of what is best for an aged relative—warmth, safety, hot meals—may not be those of the old person himself. He—more likely she—might prefer risking a fall in a cold kitchen and dying of hypothermia to the most luxurious nursing home or to moving in with a son or daughter in an unfamiliar area away from friends.

Serious dementia is, of course, a different matter and increasingly common; in-patient care may be the only option. Such people have become mentally impaired and the relationship of professionals who care for them is very similar to that which exists with other mentally handicapped adults. Their dignity is of great importance, but many decisions have to be taken on their behalf and the questions of when to treat and when to investigate rest even more firmly on the shoulders of the doctor. A demented person may not necessarily be unhappy, and may have an inner life not detectable to the outsider.

Terminally ill patients in another age group, such as a younger person with a malignant disease, often have their lives legitimately shortened by the adequate administration of powerful pain-relieving drugs; the principle of double effect is suitably applied in such a case. Demented old people rarely require such drugs, so that a decision to allow them to die will usually involve the withholding of specific treatment for intercurrent illness. Decisions concerning which therapeutic means are appropriate in each case are a matter for precise medical and nursing judgment.

While too many of the trappings of hospital care are undesirable and distasteful both for the dying person and the family, a catheter in the bladder may be much more comfortable and unobtrusive than the constant need to change wet bed linen; an intravenous saline drip into the back of the hand is discreet and unencumbering and will relieve any distressing symptoms of dehydration in a febrile patient. These measures make dying more comfortable without significantly affecting the outcome and detract nothing from the dignity we all desire at the end.

The compassion and skill of the hospice staff enable dying people to participate in the management of their own dying. Most of us, however, die in less well-ordered circumstances, of diseases associated with growing old. Old people too need help actively to disengage from former activities and responsibilities and to prepare for the time when they must let go altogether and say "into thy hands."

Euthanasia

This subject generates much heat in general discussion, but it has been my experience in ordinary life and in family medical practice that the question is quite rarely encountered.

"Euthanasia" is here being used in its modern and more usual sense of the direct termination of a patient's life at her specific request in the face of an illness she is finding intolerable. Its literal sense of a good or easy death is no more than we would all wish for, something that should be offered by good terminal care. Allowing a person to die by standing back and allowing nature to take its course has already been discussed and is part of good and well-judged professional care. It is sometimes referred to as "passive euthanasia," but this seems to me to be a needlessly confusing term.

Many patients facing terminal illness will ask overtly or circumspectly to be assured that they will be kept as free as possible from distress and pain. When the end is in sight they or their family may make it explicitly clear that they would prefer adequate sedation to a few extra days of dying. In such circumstances the morality of the principle of double effect is rarely questioned by either patient or doctor. It is not even customary to enter sedation as a contributory cause of death on the death certificate, though it is certain that this has often been the case.

Patients with malignant disease may have been receiving high doses of strong analgesics by the end. Hospice-type management is spreading rapidly in the community and a woman with cancer of the breast, for example, which has spread to the bone, may be started and maintained comfortably on oral diamorphine while continuing to play a reasonably active role in family life. Large doses are not necessary at first if correctly administered with the patient's cooperation, but they are of course stepped up if the need increases and tolerance possibly develops.

Powerful drugs should never be withheld for reasons of medical timidity; the dosage should always be governed by the patient's needs. Correct combinations of analgesic drugs used in conjunction if necessary with specific nerve-blocking techniques can allow most patients to be both reasonably alert and pain free; confidence that their needs will be met is a very important factor in maintaining their morale. There is nothing more distressing than to see a patient dying in a general hospital that is no longer suitable for her needs. She anxiously watches the clock waiting for the statutory four hours to pass before she will be "due" for another injection. Hospice methods have overcome this problem and deserve high praise.

Emphysema is a common and distressing condition frequently met in family practice and is much more difficult to handle. It is often the late result of chronic bronchitis, where the actual alveolar lung tissue has been destroyed. It is in these air spaces that oxygenation of the blood takes place and sufferers are chronically short of breath. In the late stages of this condition, the patients use all the accessory muscles of respiration to inflate the remaining lung tissue to the full; they literally have to sit up and stay awake to breathe. They are not in pain but simple sedatives to encourage sleep are ineffective for the foregoing reason. Oxygen from a cylinder helps a little, but terminally such patients are in a very pitiable condition. Morphine is the only drug that gives real relief by diminishing the actual body cell requirement for oxygen, but there is no doubt that even in a small dose it will reduce the respiratory drive and directly hasten death.

Whether, and when, to administer morphine to such a patient calls for considerable medical judgment and even courage. It is probably in treating cases of respiratory distress that most family doctors come nearest to practicing euthanasia.

In this doctors must be clear. To hasten a patient's end by deliberate action, even by a few days, is legally regarded as murder. The category of "mercy killing" does not exist, at least in British law, though a court might be expected to reduce a charge to manslaughter. Ethically, and therefore most importantly, it would seem that the *intention* of the doctor is the overriding factor. Most people would consider that there is a clear moral difference between an actual intention to kill and taking even the admittedly high risk of administering a powerful sedative to a patient in respiratory distress with the primary intention of giving that person a night's rest. Such action would be most unlikely to come to court and I have no doubt that it is widely practiced.

Persistent Vegetative State

In hospital practice there is the substantial legal and ethical problem of caring for patients who are in a permanent coma from irreversible cortical brain damage but whose lower brain is still functioning so that they can breathe without a ventilator—the so-called persistent vegetative state (PVS). The diagnosis of cortical death by electro-encephalography is discussed in the next chapter (transplant surgery), but these criteria apply only to those whose conventional signs of life—spontaneous heartbeat and respiration—have ceased. Those unfortunate patients in PVS are cortically dead but they are not dead by the usually accepted standards; it would be unthinkable, for instance, to bury a person whose heart was still beating.

Since they are unconscious and have lost the swallowing reflex they must be tube-fed. Civil law hinges on whether this constitutes "normal nursing care" or, to use the moral language of the church, on whether it involves "ordinary or extraordinary means" of treatment.

The patient who is reliably diagnosed as being in PVS has no self-regarding interests so there is no patient-based reason to continue life-sustaining treatments, including artificial hydration and nutrition.[4]

The code of practice of the British Medical Association draws a distinct line between withholding drugs or nutrition, and administering a drug to allow a patient to die. The civil law varies from country to country and from state to state. At the time of writing, American courts have acceded to families' requests in around 80 cases, ruling that life-sustaining treatment could be discontinued. Withdrawal of tube-feeding and hydration in these circumstances is licit in Scotland insofar as it is understood that the law will not concern itself in cases where the doctor has made his decision in good faith after seeking a second opinion and consulting the family. I personally support this position; unconscious people do not suffer from hunger or thirst and any restlessness could be controlled by sedation. This person cannot live a meaningful life, and the strain on the near relatives is unjustified and cruel.

In England the legal position is unresolved and a doctor acting on her own judgment would lay herself open to a possible charge of murder. As a result it has been estimated that a possible 1000-1200 patients in PVS are currently being kept alive at the cost of great mental suffering to the relatives and several million pounds annually to the National Health Service. An appeal was filed in September 1992 on behalf of the parents of a young man still lying unconscious in a hospital from brain injury sustained in a soccer stadium disaster in April 1989. The appeal was allowed two months later, but awaits ratification.

With regard to the general question of legalizing euthanasia, it is widely reported that the majority of the lay public both in Europe and the United States supports the provision of *positive* help toward a rapid and peaceful death. This is generally understood to entail the administration of a lethal injection. If such a procedure were to be legalized the immediate question would arise as to who would carry this out. I know of no survey of medical opinion on the matter but I would expect that many if not most doctors would regard such legislation as gravely threatening to undermine that trust between patient and physician which is central to medical practice and enshrined in every professional code.

Chapter 11

TRANSPLANT SURGERY

Kidney transplant is now a well established procedure to which few people have any ethical objection. In the early years, even when related donors were used, the problems of tissue matching and rejection were very great, but many of these difficulties have been overcome and there is now a high expectation of success. The fact that we have two kidneys makes live donation possible and in some centers, notably in Scandinavia, cadaveric transplant is almost a thing of the past. While donating a kidney is hardly analogous to giving a pint of blood, the danger to the donor that the other kidney might fail is considerably less than 0.1 percent. The advantages of live donation are of course enormous. Not only is the kidney absolutely fresh but tissue matching has been confirmed without haste and the operation arranged well in advance so that the recipient, who is probably on dialysis several times a week, is both physically and psychologically prepared. In the case of cadaver donation, the midnight telephone call to alert patient and transplant team places a tremendous strain on both recipient and hospital. Live donation of a kidney to some young relative in renal failure is thus an act of admirable and usually rewarding charity.

A cadaveric kidney must be removed quickly after death if it is to be useful. The word "donor" is, of course, a euphemism for a young person who has most likely been killed in an accident. Obtaining consent, therefore, almost inevitably involves approaching a bereaved family while they are still shocked and distressed. The suggestion has been made in Britain that the law should be changed to presume consent unless otherwise stated.[1]

People fail to carry organ donation cards more often through inertia than considered opposition, and it seems reasonable to expect that many lives could be saved if the law could be changed in this way.

In the last five years successes have been reported using pigs' kidneys. This may represent a major breakthrough and unless there is an objection to killing animals for any reason whatsoever, including food, there seems to me to be no substantial ethical problem. Pigs' heart valves have been used in cardiac surgery for several years and "catgut"—usually sheep's gut—sutures have been used in routine surgery for decades because of their absorbable quality. Many people who will not eat meat for humanitarian reasons wear leather shoes or play a musical instrument with gut strings. If there is an objection it would have to be a consistent one.

The Diagnosis of Death

I said earlier that the diagnosis of death is usually easy. The development of sophisticated ventilatory techniques for patients in a coma from brain injury provide circumstances in which this statement does not apply. Body cells die at different rates; the brain cells are least able to withstand anoxia and die first, while those of skin, nails, and hair follicles may live for one or two days longer. The term "brain death" has become popular with the lay public, but brain cells too die at different rates: the cortical cells first, then the thalamus, and last the brain-stem which includes the respiratory center. It is thus necessary to make a distinction between human life and biological life. Human life is associated with cortical activity and viability of cortical cells can be demonstrated by electroencephalography. A flat response after standard stimulation procedures is usually taken to mean the end of human life and this test, repeated and confirmed by more than one doctor, is normally taken as an indication of turning off the life-support system, if there is one. It should be noted that in human terms the patient is dead *before* the machine is switched off, a point which many people fail to grasp and which is the source of much natural anxiety.

If it is planned to use the organs for transplant after cortical death has been established there are several alternatives open to the transplant team after finding and preparing a suitable tissue-matching recipient. If the ventilator is stopped the respiratory center in the brain stem will quickly die from lack of oxygen. The heart is less susceptible to anoxia than the brain and is likely to continue to beat for some minutes until it too runs out of oxygen. After cessation of the heartbeat the patient is dead by conventional as well as neurological standards and the required organs are removed as soon as possible for immediate transfer, freezing, or perfusion. So that the organs remain in good condition the donor must already have been moved to the vicinity of an operating theater before the ventilator is stopped. For the sake of the relatives it would seem best that they should be informed that the patient is dead as soon as it has been confirmed and that the time given on the certificate of death should relate to this moment.

Heart Transplant

Live donation of single vital organs is, of course, by definition impossible. Cadaveric liver transplant is as yet less successful than that of the kidney but the many technical and rejection problems are being overcome. Heart transplant is not only the most dramatic but the one that evokes the greatest emotional response. This should cause little surprise since the heart has been perceived for so long in history and in literature as the source and essence of life and personhood. It is true, though, that "from the biological point of view a transplanted heart is less apt to injure the spiritual personality of the recipient than are certain accepted psychiatric and neurosurgical techniques."[2]

Since the circulatory system works on the ordinary principles of hydrodynamics and the heart is merely the pumping machine, the same comment could apply to a mechanical or animal heart if such a thing were to become a practical possibility.

The main ethical problem in doing a heart transplant seems to be in justifying such elaborate procedures to prolong the life of a person whose expectation of life is in any case poor. It is unlikely to be considered unless the recipient's heart is in intractable failure; in such circumstances the secondary effect of cardiac failure on other organs may already be severe and irreversible. The postoperative mortality is high and the most that can be hoped for in most cases is a very few years of survival. Heart transplant in newborns seems to be particularly questionable. Even if it is successful the problem of growth has to be dealt with. Will the heart grow with the baby and what will be the effect of immunosuppressive drugs on the baby's own growth? Because something *can* be done, it does not necessarily mean that it *should* be done.

The whole problem lies in the difficult area of balancing the particular against the common good. If the money spent on heart transplant were to be used to fund a heart-disease prevention program or to reduce the waiting time for simpler, more successful heart operations—coronary bypass or the correction of some valvular defects—there is no doubt that the common good would be better served. That kind of problem is, however, encountered by all of us in daily living. The only practicable guide is probably the old wisdom that you must do what you can, but do only what you *can* do. If I am a doctor I must devote my skill to the treatment of each individual patient with heart disease. If I am a health commissioner or engaged in the administration of public resources, I will devote my energy to improving the nutritional balance of school children's meals and discourage cigarette smoking.

The Beating Heart Donor

Since organs begin to deteriorate immediately after their blood supply stops, the "beating heart donor" (who is cortically dead) is an alternative and logical source of transplant material, although it must be stated that there are transplant surgeons as well as many members of the public who are unable to accept this.

The argument for the procedure on purely biological and utilitarian grounds is irrefutable. If the organs are to be donated, it is reasonable to ensure that they are in the best possible condition; there can be no more efficient way of achieving this than to maintain the heart and circulation by keeping the donor on the respirator and continuing to ventilate the lungs until the recipient is surgically prepared. The donor has been pronounced cortically and therefore humanly dead and simple ventilation of the lungs is more efficient and effective than any heart-lung machine or perfusion apparatus that could be substituted in an operating theater. The donor's body *is*, in effect, a biological heart-lung-perfusion machine.

The arguments against beating-heart donation must therefore be on a different plane. Some surgeons instinctively recoil from the idea, even though they know the standard tests for death have been applied and the criteria fulfilled. Others who do not, and consider the recipient's needs to be paramount, may nevertheless clear the operating theater of nurses and auxiliary staff to spare their feelings until the donor heart has been removed and the body taken out of the operating room. It has been suggested that a general anesthetic could be given in case there should be pain, but this is not reassuring.

For the relatives of the donor it asks a degree of super-human scientific detachment, which can be by no means assumed in the emotional circumstances of the death of a young person. However well the relatives may have been prepared it may seem humanly inappropriate to deny them a time of quiet leave taking, free from the background noise and impedimenta of the life support system. It is possible too that the lamentably small number of people who carry organ donation cards would diminish even further if they thought their organs might be taken before they were "really" dead.

While the recipients would undoubtedly gain, it is an area where utilitarian considerations are not necessarily supreme and provides yet another example of the difficulty of discerning in any given situation who is one's neighbor.

The Fetus as Donor

There was considerable disquiet as well as interest in 1988 when it was reported that the transplant of brain tissue from a dead fetus had benefitted a patient with Parkinson's disease.

The term "stillborn" is applied to a baby born after the 28th week of pregnancy who has "not breathed or shown other signs of life." In most societies it is customary for the parents of the child to arrange for burial or cremation. The stillborn infant is generally regarded as the property of its parents and their permission is required before any of its organs or tissues can be used for donation or experiment. In the UK the "28 weeks" is a relic of the Infant Life (Preservation) Act of 1929, and since babies more premature than this may now survive, it is clearly no longer appropriate. It must be remembered too that gestational age is never more than an approximation, so that "breathing and other signs of life" are more important factors than prematurity per se. A premature infant born at 26 weeks that succumbed after a week would be considered like any other baby to have "died." Previable and incomplete fetuses have been, for practical purposes, long regarded as discarded biological material and although the mother would have the right to refuse permission, they have traditionally been available for research or teaching purposes. Outside of university hospitals and research centers it is customary to dispose of them by incineration.

In the case of anencephaly the status of the fetus as a "brain-dead donor" is unclear as the normal criteria for brain death cannot be applied. The question is not yet resolved in the UK or in the United States, although donation is permitted in Germany.

The Christian churches, including the Catholic church, do not seem, in practice, to have clear-cut procedures for either baptism or burial of a previable or non-viable fetus, and although a mother will grieve over a spontaneous abortion or miscarriage she tends, in my experience, to have neither curiosity nor strong feelings about the physical disposal of the conceptus. There is no doubt that a great deal of useful study has been and is being carried out on fetal tissue set aside for this purpose.

If there is an ethical problem in respect of fetal tissue for transplant procedures, it must hinge on the question of whether it arises from an abortion that was spontaneous or induced. In either case, the conceptus once separated from the mother is dead. The considerations are in some ways similar to those that apply to the 14-day embryo and the legitimacy of experimentation upon it. A moral distinction has been made by some churches between those embryos that are adventitiously available as a by-product of IVF and those that might be produced for the express purpose of experimentation (VS). The embryos are indistinguishable biologically and are equally useful. The dead embryo or fetus from a spontaneous abortion or miscarriage is similarly indistinguishable from that produced as a result of active termination of pregnancy; both are common, however regrettable that may be.

In view of the wide availability of these fetuses, it seems to me to be unduly alarmist to suggest that the use of fetal tissue for transplant or research might lead to inducing women to breed and abort fetuses expressly for the purposes, or that a neurosurgeon would actively persuade a gynecological colleague to terminate a pregnancy in order to provide him or her with a fetal brain tissue.

It is difficult, if not impossible to take a general moral stand on transplant surgery. Each procedure has a difficult ethical content, and while kidney transplant seems virtually free of moral problems it too can be open to abuse. Cases have been reported of poor people in Latin America or the Middle East selling one of their kidneys to a rich recipient. While the use of the "beating heart donor" may seem instinctively to some to be a distasteful procedure, there are others who would claim that a desperately ill recipient has an overriding claim.

Human organs do not have the status of a human person, but it is important that the considerations of human dignity and public disquiet should never be brushed aside or disregarded.

Chapter 12

The Harm We Do

The dispensing of both drugs and advice is a tricky procedure and of particular concern perhaps to the family doctor who has a patient in her long-term care and may enjoy a degree of personal trust and confidence not shared by a hospital department. She has the traditional authority to "certify" whether or not a patient is fit for work, for life insurance, or to decide whether some complaint merits referral for further investigation.

Doctors in general know more than their patients about bodily health and disease, so much of their authority is reasonably derived from their specialized knowledge. There is a danger, however (which applies equally to the minister or priest), that too much paternalistic authority in the doctor might be *encouraged* by patients and become a substitute for the more difficult task of ordering their own lives wisely. A balance has to be struck between discouraging overdependence on doctors and adopting a false sense of equality that would deny doctors any authority whatsoever and render them professionally ineffective.

To the medical practitioner, the moral principle *"primum non nocere"*—"above all, do no harm"—does not mean that one should never inflict or risk harm at all. Medical practice is unthinkable without a willingness to risk harm to patients. It means, rather, that any harm risked or inflicted would have to be justified by a reasonable expectation of benefits.[1]

Patients cannot themselves be expected to balance the therapeutic usefulness of any drug against its possible side effects, even when they have been told what these might be. Most doctors will have seen a patient become seriously anemic, for example, from taking aspirin-related drugs prescribed for a rheumatic disorder. Although they have been properly warned about possible digestive discomfort, they might well fail to recognize the insidious symptoms of slow gastro-intestinal bleeding.

If, on the other hand, too much is made of the possible adverse effects of a really beneficial or even life-saving drug, the patient might be reluctant to give it a chance.

Unusually far-reaching side effects are illustrated by the following case.

A woman was referred through a national counseling agency on account of marital difficulties. Seven years earlier her husband had planned to retire from work at 55 so that they could enjoy their good health and comfortable pension. They had greatly looked forward to this, planning to move to the country and to explore Europe. A few months before his retirement her husband had had a minor coronary thrombosis, which entailed only a few days in the hospital. He had been reassured that the damage was minimal and had been put on some "tablets," which he was still taking. Unfortunately, his wife said, he had never really recovered. He went back to work until his 55th birthday but since this short illness he had lost all his normal energy and enthusiasm for life. Worst of all, he had become impotent and since their physical marital relations had always been warm, this had caused them great concern and perplexity. He was ashamed and embarrassed, refusing to discuss it with her or anyone else and they had generally stopped making any demonstration of affection to each other. The car was sold and the new house became a disaster since he had neither the energy nor inclination to look after the garden. She was bitterly disappointed at the way their later years had turned out after a very happy marriage, and she was almost suicidally depressed.

On tactful inquiry it was found that the "heart tablets" the husband was taking were beta-blockers, which act by chemically blocking nerve receptors in the heart muscle, thereby reducing its work and its demand for oxygen. The value of this group of drugs in coronary artery disease and hypertension is unquestioned; severe anginal pain can be well controlled, but reduced cardiac output means a diminished response to exercise, with consequent breathlessness and fatigue. A direct side effect in the male may be sexual impotence, as in this man's case. This man had been taking the drug for many years with doubtful therapeutic benefit to his heart. Adjustment to retirement can be difficult in any case, but with this man, lethargy, and particularly impotence, had almost certainly led to secondary psychological effects that virtually destroyed his retirement and a happy marriage.

The presenting problem to the counselor was severe depression in his wife but it was eventually traced back to ill-advised, long-term medication that had been given to her husband without adequate explanation. Although the medication was subsequently discontinued, the damage to their relationship had already been done.

Beta-blockers also affect other nerve receptors that trigger the body's response to nervous stress and may be used in place of some of the more discredited tranquilizing drugs, since they relieve the symptoms of stress without the danger of sedation or addiction.

They are often used by musicians, for example, as a single small dose before a performance. In these circumstances they prevent the bodily symptoms of acute short-lived stress such as palpitation, sweating, and tremor, while not interfering with mental acuity and neuro-muscular function. Sweating and tremor of the hands can seriously interfere with playing a musical instrument, and the occasional use of this group of drugs in such circumstances appears to be justifiable and harmless.

If beta-blockers are used for the relief of stress over a long period, it is most important that the patient clearly understands what the adverse effects might be so that they are promptly recognized.

Historically, people have always looked for relief from stress, the oldest agent probably being alcohol. Opiates, barbiturates, and more recently the benzodiazapenes have all been in vogue, but have now been discarded because of their many drawbacks.

The major tranquilizing and anti-depressant drugs are of immense value in the treatment of serious psychotic disorders, and many people with chronic mental illness are able to live a reasonably normal life with the help of appropriate medication.

A short use of anti-depressants will probably curtail a less serious but unpleasant illness like post-viral depression, but the following case illustrates what might go wrong through accident or misunderstanding on the part of either doctor or patient.

A man of 61, recently retired from work, had become depressed after a bout of flu and had been started by his doctor on a tricyclic anti-depressant. About a month later he moved to a different area and had to consult a new doctor about difficulty in emptying his bladder; since he had a moderately enlarged prostate he was referred to hospital for prostatectomy. This did not relieve his symptoms, which depressed him still further, and his anti-depressants were increased. After about two years on this higher dose he was slow in speech and thought, overweight, and an old man in every way. Fortunately he moved again and his new doctor suspected that his sluggishness and urinary problems were due to over-medication with anti-depressant drugs. These were gradually reduced and eventually stopped. He lost his weight and bladder problems and regained his previous physical and mental energy.

The following case is an example of how mistaken clinical assessment coupled with unquestioned authoritarianism can gravely harm a patient's life.

A man of 45 was in good health but recited the history of a

heart murmur that had been detected on routine examination while he was at school. On account of this, his parents had been told that he must never be allowed to overexert himself and they had conscientiously excluded him from all games and other strenuous activities. Fortunately he had been admitted to the hospital at the age of 40 for minor surgery and the murmur had been noted by the anesthetist, who referred him for cardiac assessment. Careful testing with modern techniques had indicated that the heart murmur had no serious significance whatsoever. Since then he led a normal fully energetic life but had always regretted the forty years when the strenuous activities he so much enjoyed had been denied him.

The great pharmacological advances that have been made in the treatment of both physical and mental illness are not to be decried; people are living longer and more comfortably because of them. This is sometimes denied by medical critics who see such claims as spurious and would relate all seeming advances in medicine to better social conditions and the natural attenuation of previously more virulent micro-organisms. Personally, I find it difficult not to be impressed by a recovery, virtually overnight, from a serious condition like acute lobar pneumonia. Pharmacologically effective drugs almost invariably have side effects, but if the disease is life-threatening, these may simply have to be tolerated. When the situation is less clear-cut, both doctor and patient must carefully weigh the expected advantages against the drawbacks. A steamroller should never be used to crack a nut.

Fortunately, excessive medical authority is declining as patients become better educated and more articulate. The media deserve much credit in this area. In the church too, since the Second Vatican Council, the role of authority has declined in the perception of the laity if not the Roman magisterium.

Although some readers will consider that moral liberty, particularly in sexual matters, has gone too far, many Catholics will have painful memories of the days when the implantation of excessive guilt was highly destructive. They will remember the humiliation of the regular confession of even the most trivial sexual "sins." Married women with many children would feel obliged to admit refusing their marital "duties" for fear of yet another baby, or their husbands to periodic abstinence or coitus interruptus for the same reason. *All* means of family limitation were firmly condemned, it must be remembered, until 1950 as frustrating the procreative purpose of marriage. Fond memories of large, poor-but-happy Catholic families are often a product of sentiment rather than reality.

Adolescents were plagued by guilt about "impure thoughts" or transient homosexual attractions, both of which were considered to be destructive to the physical as well as the spiritual health. Excessive anxiety about these matters undermined the psychological well-being of many seminarians in particular and laid the ground for future neuroses or abandonment of the priestly vocation.

On a more general level there is no doubt that the church's historical and sustained opposition to contraception contributed significantly to the horrors of the Irish potato famine, for example, in the last century and in our time to the widespread starvation we are witnessing in countries that have overrun their food supply.

Advice can be as damaging as drugs and in this area the clergy have to be as careful as the doctors. Misguided spiritual counseling or harsh judgment of a penitent can cause, in a sensitive person, a drop in self-esteem from which they may never recover. Anxious people are acutely sensitive to tone of voice. Mistaken assessment of an isolated sinful act or a single personality weakness can cripple spiritually as the wrong interpretation of a single physical abnormality can cripple physically.

The responsibility is heavy on the shoulders of those who deal with people who are ill or in trouble, but they must never forget their human limitations.

They are not Gods
though they would like to be;
they are only a human
trying to fix up a human.[2]

Many of the dilemmas discussed in this book have resulted from comparatively recent medical advances, each of which has raised a new set of moral problems to which there are no ready answers. The Christian doctor must often be prepared, therefore, to carry the cross of uncertainty when trying to balance the needs of the particular patient against those arising from her concept of traditional Christian moral norms. In the case of the Catholic doctor, it may be from those arising from specific magisterial directions.

Until the introduction of the sulphonamides in the mid-1930s and the antibiotics a few years later, there was no question about whether an old person should be *allowed* to die from bronchopneumonia; they simply died. All babies with spina bifida quickly succumbed to meningitis, but assessing the suitability for an operation today is painful and difficult for both surgeon and parent. The severest degrees of birth defect can be diagnosed ante-natally and may constitute legal grounds for termination of pregnancy.

In the last 15 years we have seen the development of kidney transplants and more recently of single vital organs such as liver and heart. Intensive-care techniques enable a patient with severe brain damage to be kept alive for long periods, sometimes leading to near miraculous recovery, but often to the difficult decision to discontinue the life-support system when brain injury is clearly irreversible. When such a decision is made, should the overriding consideration be for the patient, for the family, or for the needs of others depending for survival on transplant of the patient's organs, after death has been confirmed? Given time to find suitable tissue-matching recipients, four lives might be saved from reception of his heart, liver, and each of his kidneys.

Contraception has been with us for centuries; primitive contraceptive devices have been found on archaeological sites and there are few household substances that have not been tried as spermicides at one time or another. It is only in our time that the doctor has become involved and success virtually guaranteed. If limiting the numbers of offspring is such an urgent human need, perhaps the time has come for the church to examine the severe strictures it has traditionally imposed. There are precedents for softening moral teaching. A good example would be the case of lying. It has been found necessary to draw a moral distinction between lying for selfish gain and "not telling the truth" to an oppressor, for example, to protect someone's safety. Could not the church maintain its stance against contraception as a license for unbridled sexual promiscuity, while allowing married couples to plan the number and spacing of their children in the manner that most enhances their dignity and well-being? After his encyclical *Humanae Vitae* in 1968, Pope Paul VI wisely accepted protest and theological dissent and it seemed for several years that the conscience of believers was to be recognized. In 1983, however, the new Code of Canon Law set out penal sanctions enforcing conformity and signified a return of the church to what has been called the sickness of legalism.

Attempts to terminate pregnancy have also been a common feature in human history, attested by the many ecclesiastic, philosophic, and legal pronouncements on the subject. Such attempts were usually made by the woman herself or by an amateur more or less skilled in the matter, and were forbidden not only by the church but by civil law. Now, however, civil law permits termination in a wide variety of circumstances. The procedures are becoming increasingly refined and are carried out in the hospital by qualified members of the medical profession whose own code of ethics in the matter closely reflects not only the law but the International Code of Medical Ethics as formulated in the Declaration of Oslo in 1970.

In the fields of infertility and genetics, particularly rapid and controversial advances are being made. While it is true that the fact that something *can* be done does not necessarily mean that it *should* be done, the benefit to infertile couples and to those with a family history of grave congenital disorder is beyond dispute. It must be said, however, that even in the best of IVF units, and even though the results are continually improving, the success rate is still only about 25 percent. For every couple who takes home a baby, three do not, and it is of the utmost importance that the patients know this from the beginning so that they are braced against the pain of failure.

Even if the church's teaching on some sexual matters may be sound at its heart, the particularity of its pronouncements has caused and is continuing to cause widespread concern. It is hard to believe today that the churches—including the Catholic church—once opposed, on moral grounds, pain relief for a woman in labor. It may be that in the next century it will seem similarly incredible that the Catholic church in our time should have prohibited the contraceptive pill.

It is right and ever more necessary that the Christian churches should concern themselves with matters relating to science and the welfare of the human race and that moral questions should be illuminated by theological insights. Laws, however, must always be at the service of values, and doctrine must always reflect the image of a loving God.

My concern in addressing these questions as a Catholic doctor and in trying to share with readers my views born of medical experience springs from a deep love of the church. I greatly fear that what it has to say on spiritual matters of central importance is becoming increasingly obscured by inappropriate moral pronouncements that endanger its credibility and marginalize those of us who are otherwise loyal and committed Catholics.

NOTES

Biblical quotations throughout the text are from the Revised Standard Version.

Introduction
1. John Mahoney, *Bio-Ethics and Belief* (London: Sheed and Ward, 1984), p. 121.

Chapter 1: Reflections on Authority
1. Walter M. Abbott, ed., *The Documents of Vatican II, Dignitatis Humanae*, sec. 2, par.3 (New York: Guild, Association, and America Presses, 1966), p. 680.

  2. *Ibid., Gaudium et Spes*, par. 62, p. 270.

  3. John Habgood, *A Working Faith* (London: Darton, Longman & Todd, 1980), p. 112.

  4. John Mahoney, *The Making of Moral Theology* (Oxford: Oxford University Press, 1987), p. 134.

  5. Habgood, *A Working Faith*, p. 114.

  6. Abbott, *Documents of Vatican II, Gaudium et Spes*, par. 16, p. 213.

Chapter 2: Some Reflections on Suffering
1. John H. Hick, *Evil & the God of Love* (London: Macmillan, 1966).

  2. Daniel Berrigan, *America Is Hard to Find* (London: SPCK, 1983).

  3. Helen Waddell, *Peter Abelard* (London: Constable, 1933), "The Paraclete."

  4. Carl Rogers, *On Becoming a Person* (Boston: Houghton Mifflin, 1961), pp. 39-44.

  5. Robert Runcie, et al., *Encounters: Exploring Christian Faith* (London: Darton, Longman & Todd, 1986), p. 9.

Chapter 3: Contraception
1. 1 Corinthians 7:6.

  2. John Mahoney, *The Making of Moral Theology*, p. 63.

  3. Mahoney, p. 63, citing *De nupt. et conc.*,2, 21, 36;PL 44, 457

  4. Mahoney, p. 62 , citing *Sermo 51, 13, 22*;PL 38, 345

  5. Jack Dominian, *Sexual Integrity* (London: Darton, Longman & Todd, 1978), p. 39.

  6. Nancy Loudon, ed., *Handbook of Family Planning* (Edinburgh: Churchill Livingston, 1991), p. 143.

  7. Sean McDonagh, *The Greening of the Church* (Maryknoll, N.Y.:Orbis Books, 1990).

8. Loudon, p. 445.
9. Loudon, pp. 445, 447.
10. Dominian, pp. 72ff.

Chapter 4: Sterilization
1. "Nothing Is Unthinkable," editorial, *The Lancet* (15 Sept. 1990) vol. 336, pp. 659ff.
2. J. K. Mason and R. A. McCall Smith, *Law and Medical Ethics*, 2nd ed. (London: Butterworth, 1987), p. 69. The authors cite the "Jeanette" case in clarifying the legal situation of a minor referred for sterilization.

Chapter 5: Christian Marriage and Sexual Relations in Handicapped People
1. The Bishops' Conferences of Great Britain, "Christian Marriage and Sexual Relationships of Disabled People," *Briefing 89* (31 March 1989) vol. 19, no. 7.

Chapter 6: The Status of the Embryo
1. Sacred Congregation for the Doctrine of the Faith, *Declaration on Abortion*, par. 1471, 1974.
2. G. R. Dunstan and Mary J. Seller (eds.), *The Status of the Human Embryo*. King Edward's Hospital Fund for London, p. 45, citing *Quaestionum in Hept.,I, II n. 80*, 1988.
3. *Ibid.*, p. 47, citing *Summa Theologiae*. 2a 2ae, 64. 1.
4. John Mahoney, *The Making of Moral Theology*, p. 9.
5. Bernard Häring, *Medical Ethics*, rev. ed. (Langley: St. Paul Publications, 1974), pp. 101-102.
6. Kenneth Boyd, Brendan Callaghan, Edward Shotter, *Life Before Birth: Consensus in Medical Ethics* (London: SPCK, 1986), p. 21. The authors cite *Abortion: An Ethical Discussion* (London: Church Information Office, 1965).
7. *Ibid.*, p. 23. The authors cite General Synod, *Report of Proceedings*, vol. 10, no. 3 (London: Church Information Office, 1979), p. 1158.
8. *Ibid.*, p. 28. The authors cite General Assembly of the Church of Scotland, *Social and Moral Welfare Report*, 1966.
9. Michael J. Coughlan, *The Vatican, the Law, and the Human Embryo* (London: Macmillan, 1990), pp. 20, 74ff.
10. Teilhard de Chardin, *The Phenomenon of Man* (Glasgow: Collins, 1959).
11. Häring, *Medical Ethics*, pp. 83-84.
12. Herbert McCabe, *God Matters* (London: Geoffrey Chapman, 1987), pp. 111, 118.
13. Edward Schillebeeckx, *The Eucharist*, 2nd ed. (London: Sheed & Ward, 1977), p. 100.

Chapter 7: Abortion
1. Alastair Campbell, *Moral Dilemmas in Medicine*, 3rd ed. (London: Churchill Livingstone, 1984), p. 126.
2. The Sacred Congregation for the Doctrine of the Faith, *Instruction in*

Respect of Human Life and the Dignity of Procreation, sec. 2, par. 2.

3. J.K. Mason, R.A. McCall Smith, *Law and Medical Ethics,* 2nd ed. (London: Butterworth, 1987), p. 83.

4. *Ibid.,* p. 83.

5. *Ibid.,* p. 69.

6. Joint Statement of the Catholic Archbishops of Great Britain, *Abortion and the Right to Life,* 1980, par. 21.

7. Report to the Catholic Bishops' Joint Committee on Bio-Ethical Issues, "Post-Coital Contraception," 1985.

Chapter 8: Infertility

1. Kenneth Boyd, Brendan Callaghan, Edward Shotter, *Life Before Birth,* pp. 87-88.

2. The Sacred Congregation for the Doctrine of the Faith, *Instruction in Respect of Human Life in Its Origin and the Dignity of Procreation,* 1987, part 2: "Interventions upon Human Procreation."

3. Boyd, Callaghan, Shotter, *Life Before Birth,* p. 96. The authors cite CIS (1983), p. 10.

4. *Ibid.,* p. 101.

5. *Ibid.,* p. 103.

6. The Sacred Congregation for the Doctrine of the Faith, *Instruction in Respect of Human Life in Its Origin and the Dignity of Procreation,* 1987, part 2: "Is Homologous IVF Morally Licit?"

7. Boyd, Callaghan, Shotter, *Life Before Birth,* p. 96. The authors cite CIS (1983), p. 10.

8. J.K. Mason, *Human Life and Medical Practice* (Edinburgh: University Press, 1988), p. 91.

9. J. K. Mason and R. A. McCall Smith, *Law and Medical Ethics,* 2nd ed., (London: Butterworth, 1987), p. 45.

10. Boyd, Callaghan, Shotter, *Life Before Birth,* pp. 7ff.

11. *Ibid.,* p. 102.

12. Brother Lawrence of the Resurrection (17th century), transl. by John J. Delaney, *The Practice of the Presence of God* (Garden City, N.Y.: Doubleday), Second Conversation, 28 September 1666, p. 43.

13. Mason and McCall Smith, *Law and Medical Ethics,* p. 45.

14. Boyd, Callaghan, Shotter, *Life Before Birth,* p. 88. The authors cite CIS (1983), p. 8.

15. *Ibid.,* p. 92. The authors cite Church of Scotland, *Reports to the General Assembly, Board for Social Responsibility,* 1985, p. 290.

16. Free Church Federal Council and British Council of Churches, *Choices in Childlessness,* London, 1982, p. 45.

17. W. J. Winslade, "Private Right or Public Wrong?" *Journal of Medical Ethics,* 1981.

Chapter 9: Homosexuality and AIDS

1. Bernard Häring, *Medical Ethics,* p. 185.

2. Robert Nugent, Jeannine Gramick, *Building Bridges: Gay and Lesbian Reality and the Catholic Church* (Mystic, Conn.: Twenty-Third Publications, 1991), p. 27.

Chapter 10: Death and Dying
1. Bernard Häring, *Manipulation* (Langley: St. Paul Publications, 1975), p. 106.
2. Mason and McCall Smith, *Law and Medical Ethics*, pp. 105-106.
3. Ivan Illich, *Medical Nemesis* (London: Calder & Boyars, 1975), pp. 40-41.
4. John M. Stanley, ed., "Developing Guidelines for Decisions to Forego Life-Prolonging Medical Treatment," Supplement to *Journal of Medical Ethics*, Sept. 1992, vol. 18, part 2, par. 13.

Chapter 11: Transplant Surgery
1. Mason and McCall Smith, *Law and Medical Ethics*, p. 228.
2. Bernard Häring, *Medical Ethics*, p. 138. Häring cites Charles Dubost, "Scientific and Ethical Problems in Organ Transplantation," *The Annals of Thoracic Surgery* (August 1962), p. 102.

Chapter 12: The Harm We Do
1. John M. Stanley, ed., *Developing Guidelines for Decisions to Forego Life-Prolonging Medical Treatment*, Supplement to the *Journal of Medical Ethics* (Sept. 1992), vol. 18, introd. notes to preamble, par. 6.
2. Alastair V. Campbell, *Moderated Love: A Theology of Pastoral Care* (London: SPCK, 1984), p. 26. Campbell cites Anne Sexton, "Doctors" in *The Awful Rowing Towards God* (Boston: Houghton-Mifflin, 1975), pp. 74ff.

BIBLIOGRAPHY

Abbott Walter M., ed. *The Documents of Vatican II*. New York: Guild, Association, and America Presses, 1966.

Berrigan, Daniel. *America Is Hard to Find*. London: SPCK, London, 1973.
Bishops' Conference of Great Britain. "Christian Marriage and Sexual Relationships of Disabled People," *Briefing* 89, no. 7, vol. 19.
Boyd, Kenneth, Brendan Callaghan, Edward Shotter. *Life Before Birth: Consensus in Medical Ethics*. London: SPCK, 1986.
Brother Lawrence of the Resurrection, transl. by John J. Delaney. *The Practice of the Presence of God*. Garden City, New York: Doubleday.

Campbell, Alastair V. *Moderated Love: A Theology of Pastoral Care*. London: SPCK, 1984.
———————. *Moral Dilemmas in Medicine*, 3rd ed. London: Churchill Livingstone, 1984.
Church of Scotland. *Report to the General Assembly*. Board for Social Responsibility, 1985.
Coughlan, Michael J. *The Vatican, the Law, and the Human Embryo*. London: Macmillan, 1990.
Curran, Charles E. *Issues in Sexual and Medical Ethics*. Notre Dame, Ind.: University of Notre Dame Press, 1978.
———————. *Faithful Dissent*. London: Sheed and Ward, 1986.

Dominian, Jack. *Sexual Integrity*. London: Darton, Longman & Todd, 1978.
Dubost, Charles. "Scientific and Ethical Problems in Organ Transplantation," *The Annals of Thoracic Surgery*. August 1969.
Dunstan, G. R. *In-Vitro Fertilization: The Ethics*. Human Reproduction, 1986.
———————. "Screening for Fetal and Genetic Abnormality: Social and Ethical Issues," *Journal of Medical Genetics*, 1988.
Dunstan, G.R., ed. *The Human Embryo: Aristotle and the Arabic and European Traditions*. Exeter: University of Exeter Press, 1990.
Dunstan, G. R. and Mary J. Seller, eds. *The Status of the Human Embryo*. King Edward's Hospital Fund for London, 1988.

Ford, Norman M. *When Did I Begin?* Cambridge: Cambridge University Press, 1988.
Free Church Federal Council and British Council of Churches. "*Choices in Childlessness*," 1982.

Greeley, Andrew. "Who Are the Catholic 'Conservatives'?" *America* September 21, 1991.

Habgood, John. *A Working Faith.* London: Darton, Longman & Todd, 1980.

Häring, Bernard. *Medical Ethics*, rev. ed. Langley: St. Paul Publications, 1974.

_____. *Manipulation.* Langley: St. Paul Publications, 1975.

Hick, John. *Evil & the God of Love.* London: Macmillan, 1966.

Illich, Ivan. *Medical Nemesis.* London: Calder & Boyars, 1975.

Joint Statement of the Catholic Archbishops of Great Britain. *Abortion and the Right to Life.* London: CTS, 1980.

Kaiser, Robert Blair. *The Encyclical That Never Was.* London: Sheed and Ward, 1985.

Kelly, Kevin. "Embryo Research: The Ethical Issues," *The Month,* February 1990.

_____. "The Embryo Research Bill: Some Underlying Ethical Issues," *The Month,* March 1990.

Kushner, Harold S. *When Bad Things Happen to Good People.* London: Pan Books, Ltd. New York: Simon and Schuster, 1982.

Lancet "Nothing Is Unthinkable," editorial. September 15, 1990.

Loudon, Nancy, ed. *Handbook of Family Planning.* Edinburgh: Churchill Livingston, 1991.

Mahoney, John. "Warnock: A Catholic Comment," *The Month,* September 1984.

_____. *Bioethics and Belief.* London: Sheed and Ward, 1984.

_____. *The Making of Moral Theology.* Oxford: Oxford University Press, 1987.

Mason, J.K. *Human Life and Medical Practice.* Edinburgh: Edinburgh University Press, 1988.

Mason, J.K. and R.A. McCall Smith. *Law and Medical Ethics.* London: Butterworth, 1987.

McCabe, Herbert. *God Matters.* London: Geoffrey Chapman, 1987.

McCormick, Richard A. "Moral Theology in the Year 2000," *America,* April 18, 1992.

McDonagh, Sean. *The Greening of the Church.* Maryknoll, N.Y.: Orbis Books, 1990.

McLean, Sheila, ed. *Legal Issues in Human Reproduction.* Brookfield, Vt.: Gower, 1990.

Noonan, John T. Jr. *Contraception.* Cambridge, Mass: Belknap Press of Harvard University Press, 1986.

Nugent, Robert, Jeannine Gramick. *Building Bridges: Gay and Lesbian Reality and the Catholic Church.* Mystic, Conn: Twenty-Third Publications, 1991.

Ranke-Heinemann, Uta. *Eunuchs for Heaven*. London: Andre Deutch, 1990.

Report to the Catholic Bishops' Joint Committee on Bio-Ethical Issues. *Post-Coital Contraception*, 1985.

Rogers, Carl. *On Becoming a Person*. Boston: Houghton Mifflin, 1961.

Runcie, Robert, et al. *Encounters: Exploring Christian Faith*. London: Darton, Longman & Todd, 1986.

Sacred Congregation for the Doctrine of the Faith. *Declaration on Abortion*, 1974.

Sacred Congregation for the Doctrine of the Faith. *Commentaries*. Washington, D.C.: U.S. Catholic Conference, 1977.

Sacred Congregation for the Doctrine of the Faith. *Instruction in Respect of Human Life and the Dignity of Procreation*, 1987.

Schillebeeckx, Edward. *The Eucharist*, 2nd ed. London: Sheed & Ward, 1977.

Sexton, Anne. "Doctors," *The Awful Rowing Toward God*. Boston: Houghton Mifflin, 1975.

Stanley, John M., ed. "Developing Guidelines for Decisions to Forego Life-Prolonging Medical Treatment," Supplement, *Journal of Medical Ethics* (Sept. 1992), vol. 18.

Sutton, Agneta. *Prenatal Diagnosis: Confronting the Ethical Issues*. London: Linacre Centre, 1990.

Teilhard de Chardin, Pierre. *The Phenomenon of Man*. Glasgow: Collins, 1959.

Waddell, Helen. "The Paraclete," *Peter Abelard*. London: Constable, 1933.

Wennberg, Robert N. *Terminal Choices*. Grand Rapids, Mich.: Eerdmans, 1989.

Winslade, W.J. "Private Right or Public Wrong?" *Journal of Medical Ethics*, 1981.

Winter, Michael. *Whatever Happened to Vatican II?* London: Sheed and Ward, 1985.

Of Related Interest...

Morality and Its Beyond
Dick Westley

Fresh insights into the meaning of morality. Encourages
a "pastoral morality" within the church.
324 pp, $8.95

Catholic Morality Revisited
Gerard S. Sloyan

For anyone who might feel confusion about the meaning
of morality and for those who teach and counsel them.
160 pp, $9.95

Redemptive Intimacy
A New Perspective for the Journey to Adult Faith
Dick Westley

A forceful challenge to today's adult who may be struggling
with issues of religion, leading to development of a deeper faith.
176 pp. $5.95

A Radical* Guide for Catholics
*rooted in the essentials of our faith
Bill Huebsch, with David Peterson

Offers a vision of Christianity related to lived reality,
with emphasis on conscience development.
224 pp, $9.95

Available at religious bookstores or from
TWENTY-THIRD PUBLICATIONS
P.O. Box 180 • Mystic, CT 06355 • 1-800-321-0411